Human Development Network
Health, Nutrition, and Population Series

Reducing Maternal Mortality

Learning from Bolivia, China, Egypt, Honduras, Indonesia, Jamaica, and Zimbabwe

Marjorie A. Koblinsky
Editor

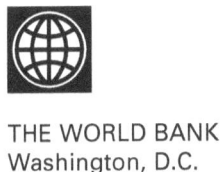

THE WORLD BANK
Washington, D.C.

© 2003 The International Bank for Reconstruction and Development / The World Bank
1818 H Street, NW
Washington, DC 20433
Telephone 202-473-1000
Internet www.worldbank.org
E-mail feedback@worldbank.org

All rights reserved.

First printing April 2003

The findings, interpretations, and conclusions expressed herein are those of the author(s) and do not necessarily reflect the views of the Board of Executive Directors of the World Bank or the governments they represent.

The World Bank does not guarantee the accuracy of the data included in this work. The boundaries, colors, denominations, and other information shown on any map in this work do not imply any judgment on the part of the World Bank concerning the legal status of any territory or the endorsement or acceptance of such boundaries.

Rights and Permissions

The material in this work is copyrighted. Copying and/or transmitting portions or all of this work without permission may be a violation of applicable law. The World Bank encourages dissemination of its work and will normally grant permission promptly.

For permission to photocopy or reprint any part of this work, please send a request with complete information to the Copyright Clearance Center, Inc., 222 Rosewood Drive, Danvers, MA 01923, USA, telephone 978-750-8400, fax 978-750-4470, www.copyright.com.

All other queries on rights and licenses, including subsidiary rights, should be addressed to the Office of the Publisher, World Bank, 1818 H Street, NW, Washington, DC 20433, USA, fax 202-522-2422, e-mail pubrights@worldbank.org.

ISBN 0-8213-5392-6
ISSN 1683-0091

Library of Congress Cataloging-in-Publication Data has been requested.

POD by LSI

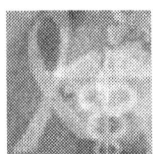

Contents

Foreword *Robert M. Hecht*	vii
Acknowledgments	xi
Acronyms and Abbreviations	xiii
Executive Summary	1
1 Factors Affecting the Reduction of Maternal Mortality *Marjorie A. Koblinsky and Oona Campbell*	5
Part 1: Case Studies	39
2 Yunnan, China, 1980–1999 *Institute for Health Science*	41
3 Honduras, 1990–1997 *Isabella Danel with Ada Rivera*	51
4 Zimbabwe, 1980–2000 *Shinga Feresu with Margaret Nyandoro and Leonard Mumbwanda*	63

Part 2: Research Studies 81

5   Bolivia, 1996–2000 83
    *Guillermo Seoane, Ramiro Equiluz,
    Miguel Ugalde, and Juan Carlos Arraya*

6   Egypt, 1992–2000 93
    Oona Campbell

7   Indonesia, 1990–1999 113
    Marjorie A. Koblinsky

8   Jamaica, 1991–1995 123
    Affete McCaw-Binns

Contributors 131

Tables

1.1	Safe Motherhood Care: Service Delivery Models	6
1.2	Changes in Delivery Care Models and Maternal Mortality Ratios	9
1.3	Factors Associated with Reduced Maternal Mortality Ratio	14
1.4	Availability of Skilled Birth Attendants	16
2.1	Huaning and Tonghai Counties, Yunnan: Maternity-Related Statistics, 1999	44
2.2	Huaning and Tonghai Counties, Yunnan: Health Care Infrastructure, 1999	46
3.1	Honduras: Referrals to Hospitals before and during Delivery, by Different Factors, 2000	56
3.2	Honduras: Referrals to Hospitals vis-à-vis Maternity Waiting Homes and Decrease in Maternal Mortality, by Different Factors, 2000	59
4.1	Zimbabwe: Select Demographic Indicators, 1962–97	65

4.2	Zimbabwe: Prevalence of HIV by Group, 1999	68
4.3	Zambia: Cause of Maternal Death, University Teaching Hospital, 1996–97	69
4.4	Zimbabwe: Number of Health Facilities, Pre-1980 and 1997	70
4.5	Zimbabwe: Infrastructure by Population Level, 1997	71
4.6	Zimbabwe: Nurses' Access Issues, 1999	73
4.7	Zimbabwe: Impact of Family Planning Program, 1984–99	75
4.8	Zimbabwe: Waiting Mothers' Shelters by Province, 1996–97	77
5.1	Bolivia: Use of Maternity Care, 1989–2000	85
5.2	Bolivia: Growth in Utilization after the National Maternal and Child Health Insurance (MCHI) Program	86
6.1	Egypt: Population-Based Studies of Maternal Mortality, 1963–2000	94
7.1	Indonesia: Assistance during Delivery, 1990, 1994, and 1997	115
7.2	South Kalimantan, Indonesia: Costs of Training Programs, 1999	117
8.1	Jamaica: Odds Ratio of Antenatal Eclampsia Cases—Intervention Parish Compared with Control Parishes, 1986–95	125
8.2	Jamaica: Number of Bed Days Used by Mothers Admitted for the Hypertensive Disorders of Pregnancy before and at the End of the Intervention Period, 1991–95	126

Figures

1.1	Determinants of Health Outcomes	12
2.1	China: Maternal Mortality Ratio and Total Fertility Rate, 1950–96	42
2.2	Huaning and Tonghai Counties, Yunnan: Hospital Delivery Rates, 1990–99	43

2.3	Yunnan: Three-Tiered Maternal and Child Health Care Network	45
4.1	Zimbabwe: Maternal Mortality Trends, 1988–99	64
4.2	Zimbabwe: AIDS, ARC, and TB Cases, 1989–96	67
4.3	Zimbabwe: Midwives by Category, 1981–97	72
6.1	Egypt: Percentage of Births by Facility and Attendant, 1976–98	95
6.2	Egypt: Percentage of Births with Cesarean Section, 1976–2000	98
6.3	Egypt: Percentage of Pregnant Women with Antenatal Care; Percentage with 4+ Visits, 1976–2000	103
6.4	Egypt: Tetanus Toxoid Immunizations during Pregnancy, 1976–2000	104
6.5	Egypt: Percentage of Women Using Modern Contraception, 1979–2001	105
7.1	South Kalimantan, Indonesia: Skill Scores for Midwives by Procedures, 1999	116
7.2	South Kalimantan, Indonesia: Skill Scores and Competency for Midwives by Groups, 1999	117
7.3	South Kalimantan, Indonesia: Proportion of Cesarean Sections among Births, 1997–99	119
7.4	South Kalimantan, Indonesia: Proportion of Births with Life-Threatening Complications in the Hospital, 1997–99	120

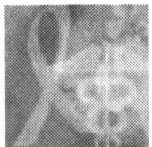

Foreword

Of the 515,000 maternal deaths that occur every year around the world, 99 percent take place in developing countries. Women in the developing world have a 1 in 48 chance of dying from pregnancy-related causes; the ratio in industrial countries is 1 in 1,800. For every woman who dies, another 30–50 women suffer injury, infection, or disease. In developing countries, pregnancy-related complications are among the leading causes of death and disability for women ages 15–49. Of all the human development indicators, the greatest discrepancy between industrial and developing countries is in maternal health.

Key interventions to improve maternal health and reduce maternal mortality are known. They include complementary, mutually reinforcing strategies: mobilizing political commitment and an enabling policy environment; investing in social and economic development such as female education, poverty reduction, and improving women's status; offering family planning services; providing quality antenatal care, skilled attendance during childbirth, and availability of emergency obstetric services for pregnancy complications; and strengthening the health system and community involvement. The challenge has been to implement these interventions in environments where political commitment, policies, and institutions and health systems have been weak. Although some countries—including very poor ones—have been successful in reducing maternal mortality, progress in many countries remains slow.

As a way to assist countries in their efforts to improve maternal health and reduce maternal mortality, we are publishing two volumes—*Investing in Maternal Health: Learning from Malaysia and Sri Lanka* and *Reducing Maternal Mortality: Learning from Bolivia, China, Egypt, Honduras, Indonesia, Jamaica, and Zimbabwe*—on success stories and lessons learned in improving health and reducing maternal mortality in a range of developing countries. The first book is based on the experiences of Malaysia and Sri Lanka during the past five to six decades. The second book discusses the more recent experiences of Bolivia, China (Yunnan), Egypt, Honduras, Indonesia, Jamaica, and Zimbabwe. These nine countries have made important strides in improving maternal health, and these books outline what worked and what did not.

The studies of maternal health in Malaysia and Sri Lanka start at a time when maternal mortality was still very high in those two countries. *Investing in Maternal Health* presents the strategies used over the past half century to reverse this situation, including maintaining a supportive policy environment and political commitment; professionalizing midwifery and ensuring skilled attendance during childbirth; strengthening health systems; introducing civil registration; and improving access to and quality of care through rural midwives with closely linked backup emergency obstetric services. Issues such as the appropriate mix of private versus public expenditures and enabling intersectoral policies are also discussed.

The case studies of Bolivia, China, Egypt, Honduras, Indonesia, Jamaica, and Zimbabwe address the issue of how maternal mortality can be reduced significantly over the course of a single decade, and which key strategies were used in these countries to achieve the reductions. These case studies also inform the current debate on whether it is wiser to invest first in skilled birth attendants, or in the care of obstetric emergencies, or both at once. The analysis also shows how strong safe motherhood policies can have an impact.

For its part, the World Bank has been strongly committed to improving maternal health and reducing maternal mortality for more than a decade and a half. The World Bank was a founding member of the Safe Motherhood Initiative in 1987 and has backed the Program of Action of the 1994 International Conference on Population and Development. More recently, the Bank has embraced the Millennium Development Goals that were agreed to in September 2000, and has made maternal health one of its top corporate priorities.

Accordingly, we hope that the experiences described in these two volumes will provide a timely contribution of hard evidence of what works as we scale up efforts to achieve the Millennium Development Goal of improving maternal health. In this sense, it is our aim that these materials help to raise the quality and effectiveness of national programs for safe motherhood backed by developing country governments and the donor community. We will endeavor, too, to ensure that the World Bank simultaneously expands its own support for this important cause.

Robert M. Hecht
The World Bank
Acting Sector Director
Health, Nutrition, and Population

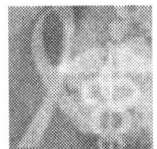

Acknowledgments

I am indebted to the many who participated in the studies—particularly the chapter authors, staff of the Ministries of Health in each country, offices of statistics, research institutes, universities, and libraries. I thank the policymakers and program managers from the present day to decades before for sharing their knowledge, experience, and insights. Providers, from referral hospitals to community-level workers, women, and families were involved in interviews or focus groups in several countries, and their insights are much appreciated. I am most grateful for the support of the John Snow, Inc. Research and Training Institute and of the donor, the World Bank.

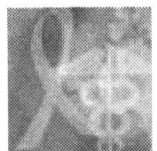

Acronyms and Abbreviations

AIDS	Acquired immune deficiency syndrome
ANC	Antenatal care
ARC	AIDS-related conditions
BDD	Bidan di desa (village-based midwife)
bEOC	Basic essential obstetric care
BHI	Basic health insurance (Bolivia)
CBD	Community-based distributors
CBR	Crude birthrate
cEOC	Comprehensive essential obstetric care
CPR	Contraceptive prevalence rate
DHS	Demographic and health surveys
ENESF	Encuesta Nacional de Epidemiología, Salud, y Fecundidad (National epidemiology and family health survey)
EOC	Essential obstetric care
ERS	Emergency Referring System
ESAP	Economic Structural Adjustment Program (Zimbabwe)
GDP	Gross domestic product
GNP	Gross national product
GP	General practitioner
HC	Health center
HIV	Human immunodeficiency virus

IEC	Information, Education and Communications programs
MCH	Maternal and child health
MCHI	National Maternal and Child Health Insurance Program (Bolivia)
MIS	Management information system
MMR	Maternal mortality ratio
MOH	Ministry of Health
MOHP	Ministry of Health and Population
MOPH	Ministry of Public Health
NGO	Nongovernmental organization
NMMS	National maternal mortality survey
OR	Odds ratio
PHC	Primary health care
RAMOS	Reproductive age mortality survey
SAM	Service Availability Module
SCM	State certified midwife
SCMN	State certified maternity nurse
SCN	State certified nurse
SMPW	Systematic management of pregnant women
SMR	Systematic management rate
SRN	State registered nurse
STD	Sexually transmitted disease
TB	Tuberculosis
TBA	Traditional birth attendant
TFR	Total fertility rate
THC	Township health center
TM	Traditional midwife
UNAIDS	Joint United Nations Program on HIV/AIDS
UNICEF	United Nations Children's Fund
USAID	U. S. Agency for International Development
UK	United Kingdom
VC	Village clinic
WHO	World Health Organization
WMS	Waiting mothers' shelters
ZNFPC	Zimbabwe National Family Planning Council

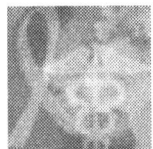

Executive Summary

The stimulus for this study was the question, Can current program strategies reduce maternal mortality more quickly than the decades required in the historically successful countries of Malaysia and Sri Lanka? The answer reached after conducting case studies and primary research on safe motherhood programs in seven countries is, no. Once a country reaches a maternal mortality ratio (MMR) of approximately 200, it can reduce its MMR by half within 7 to 10 years, as did Malaysia and Sri Lanka. However, the challenges are somewhat different for health systems today than during the 1950s–70s, when these two countries achieved an MMR of less than 100 per 100,000 live births. Lessons learned concern six factors associated with recent success in reducing mortality (Egypt; Honduras; and Yunnan, China) or with their programmatic progress toward this goal (Bolivia, Indonesia, Jamaica, and Zimbabwe).

The factor common to all the reviewed programs is the high availability of a provider who is either a skilled birth attendant or closely connected with a capable and acceptable referral system. In all countries except China, this provider has been trained to manage complications or stabilize and refer women with more severe complications. In China, the village doctors (upgraded barefoot doctors) who have not received such training have the means to refer women in need: a system for referral is relatively close by and is well linked through contractual arrangements.

A second common factor is the high availability of facilities that can provide basic and essential obstetric care. As with the skilled birth attendants, the ratio of these facilities to population is typically higher than the World Health Organization's recommended levels, and in some cases, such as in Honduras, Indonesia, and Zimbabwe, birthing centers or maternity waiting homes augment the standard health facilities. This high level of coverage with both facilities and skilled birth attendants is consistent with the findings in the historically successful countries, Malaysia and Sri Lanka.

Unlike these historic successes, however, strong government policy now focuses explicitly on safe motherhood and sets the tone for programs in all but one country, Egypt. "Access to all" had been the driving force in health care reform in Malaysia and Sri Lanka; safe motherhood had benefited along with other health programs, most likely because the midwife was the backbone of these broad health initiatives.

Another difference between the places in the present case studies and the historically successful countries is the financing of services. While services were free to families in Malaysia and Sri Lanka, costs of safe motherhood services can now be substantial and a major deterrent to use. Remedies to reduce cost, such as insurance, have proved only partially successful. Bolivia's insurance program has been helpful in increasing use of maternal services, but many of the poor remain outside the health care system. In Indonesia, one small study found that the social safety net employed there to reduce costs of services to the poor did not result in increased use of health facilities at all. Even when costs are diminished or eliminated, other barriers, such as cultural differences in birthing and distance, continue to plague the system.

A functioning referral system is considered a necessary element of safe motherhood programs, but information confirming its implementation and use can be difficult to find. Triggers to initiate referral, at the family and care provider levels, were implemented in Honduras (risk assessment) and Jamaica (cards with photos of complications) and are associated with increased appropriate use at the referral level.

The main conclusions are described further in the introductory chapter.

In summary, reduction of maternal mortality has now become an explicit focus of many programs. Where reduction is targeted and strategies are adapted to address the local barriers to use, success in moving women into appropriate care for birth has resulted, and in some cases, this has affected the reported maternal mortality. Substantial progress in a reduced maternal mortality ratio in three of the case studies was witnessed within a decade.

CHAPTER 1

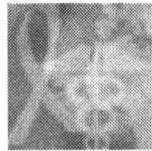

Factors Affecting the Reduction of Maternal Mortality

Marjorie A. Koblinsky and Oona Campbell

Nearly half of all maternal deaths in developing countries occur during labor or delivery, or in the immediate postpartum period. Key factors influencing programs aimed at reducing these deaths are who delivers the woman and where she delivers. A previous review of developing countries that successfully reduced maternal mortality to fewer than 100 deaths per 100,000 live births identified four basic models for implementing delivery care (Koblinsky, Campbell, and Heichelheim 1999) (see table 1.1). The models range from home delivery by a nonprofessional (including delivery in a woman's own home or in a relative's home by a traditional birth attendant, another community worker with brief health training, a relative, or alone) to delivery in a referral facility with comprehensive essential obstetric care (cEOC) by a professional skilled attendant (for example, an obstetrician or a midwife). The case studies focused on rural China, Malaysia, and Sri Lanka, places that successfully reduced maternal mortality using Models 1, 2, and 3, although reference is made to the many industrial and middle-income countries that reduced maternal mortality using Model 4 (table 1.1).

Analysis of these historical successes provides the following insights into factors affecting maternal mortality:

- Success in Model 1 (home delivery with a nonprofessional) is the exception, not the rule. Maternal mortality is staggeringly high in

Table 1.1 Safe Motherhood Care: Service Delivery Models

MODEL	REQUIRED FACTORS OF SERVICE DELIVERY	MATERNAL MORTALITY RATIOS BY LOCATION (DEATHS PER 100,000 LIVE BIRTHS)
Model 1 Nonprofessional delivery at home	• Appropriate normal birth care • Nonprofessional recognizes complications • Access to EOC organized by family or nonprofessional • Functioning EOC available	Forteleza, Brazil (1984): 120 Rural China (1996): 115
Model 2 Skilled attendant delivery at home	• Above factors, but substituting skilled birth attendant for nonprofessional	Malaysia (1970–80s): 50
Model 3 Skilled attendant delivery in basic EOC facility (health center)	• Skilled birth attendant recognizes complications; provides basic EOC in health facility • Facility organizes access to EOC • Functioning EOC available	Malaysia (1985–90s): 43 Netherlands (1983–92): 7 Sri Lanka (1996): 60
Model 4 Skilled attendant delivery in comprehensive EOC facility (hospital)	• Skilled attendant recognizes complications • Skilled attendant provides basic and comprehensive EOC	Mexico City (1988): 114 United Kingdom (1992–95): 10 United States (1990–95): 12

Note: EOC = essential obstetric care.
Sources: Koblinsky, Campbell, and Heichelheim 1999; WHO, UNICEF, and UNFPA 2001.

most places where women give birth at home with a nonprofessional. Yet nearly half of all women in developing countries do so. Even in the successful cases, rural China and a project in Forteleza, Brazil, there is no evidence that the minimally trained village doctors (community workers) or traditional birth attendants (TBAs) can reduce the maternal mortality ratio (MMR) to below 100.

- Assistance at birth by a skilled birth attendant in the home or any health facility, supported by a functioning referral system (Models 2 through 4), can reduce the MMR to around 50 or below.

Unfortunately, there is little evidence to help determine the most cost-effective of these three models, although we believe that Model 4 with specialists and highly equipped facilities is the most expensive.

- Deliveries conducted in the home (Models 1 and 2) can be successful if the health system, beginning with the referral hospital, provides outreach support to home birth attendants, whether they are traditional birth attendants, community workers, or skilled midwives. A referral and supervisory link is created from the referral facility to the home birth attendant.

- Since in Model 3—in which women are drawn into health facilities where skilled attendants give delivery care—the facility provides only basic essential obstetric care (bEOC), success depends upon links with a referral setting to address serious complications requiring blood transfusion or surgery.

- In successful Models 1 through 3, strong government policies usually guide the system of delivery care, linking the levels so that complicated cases can be, and are, referred. Service costs, and in some cases transport costs, have been free to the client, alleviating financial barriers to accessing care. Government policy often aims to ensure equitable coverage of health care.

- The assumption that Model 4, which provides comprehensive EOC, offers the "best and safest" care possible is not always borne out: studies in Mexico City and Romania have shown MMRs of greater than 100 per 100,000 despite the fact that the majority of women delivered in referral facilities (Bobadilla, Reyes, and Karchmer 1996; Stephenson and others 1992). Costs are usually higher in Model 4 than Model 3 and may be borne by the consumer.

- Once demand for delivery care at a health facility exists, women usually deliver in referral hospitals (Model 4). Health facilities without cesarean section capability, as in Model 3 settings, are typically bypassed, often because they do not have the 24-hour coverage needed for delivery care. The exception to this may be that where private sector provision is high, more use is made of Model 3 settings. In many places, the seeking of care at Model 4 settings is generally not overseen or planned by the government; rather, the consumer chooses the facility. Reversing the trend toward expensive Model 4 settings is difficult but can be achieved, as it was in Lusaka, Zambia (Murray and others 2001).

The three places whose successes provide these lessons—rural China, Malaysia, and Sri Lanka—took decades to reduce their maternal mortality. The details of their achievements are explored elsewhere (Koblinsky, Campbell, and Heichelheim 1999; Liljestrand and Pathmanathan 2002). Important questions do remain: Can countries successfully reduce MMRs to fewer than 100 per 100,000 live births more rapidly than has been reported to date? What have safe motherhood programs that act vigorously to lower maternal mortality achieved?

To address these questions, we commissioned case studies in seven new settings. These include the following:

- Three that have achieved an MMR of approximately 100 or below in the past decade—Egypt, Honduras, and Yunnan (China)

- Three that are intervening aggressively to lower maternal mortality—Bolivia, with its nationwide insurance covering care from pregnancy through the postpartum period for the mother; Indonesia, with its skilled midwife at the village level; and Jamaica, with its specific interventions aimed at reducing eclampsia deaths, its biggest killer of pregnant women

- A setting with a relatively low MMR for its geographic region—Zimbabwe (1990), which is now showing a change in that success.

Table 1.2 looks at the past and present organization of the delivery care within these seven settings, based on the models' framework, the MMRs, and the change in the MMR if available. Essentially, the changes include the following:

Table 1.2 Changes in Delivery Care Models and Maternal Mortality Ratios

MODEL CHANGES	COUNTRY	YEAR	MMR	CHANGE IN MMR (PERCENT)	SOURCE
1 to 3, 4	Bolivia	1994	390	—	INE and MI 1998
1 to 2, 3, 4	Egypt	1992–93	174		MOH 1994
		2000	84	−52	MOH 2001
1 to 4	Honduras	1990	182		Danel 1999
		1997	108	−41	
1 to 2	Indonesia	1994	390		CBS and others 1995
		1997	334	−14	CBS and others 1998
Improved 3, 4	Jamaica	1986–87	115	—	Keeling and others 1991
1 to 3, 4	Yunnan, China	1989	149		Institute of Health Sciences
		1999	101	−32	2001
3	Zimbabwe	1994	283		CSO and MI 1995
		1999	695	+245	CSO and MI 1999

— Not available.

- Indonesia is transitioning from having women deliver primarily with traditional birth attendants (Model 1) to using skilled midwives in the home (Model 2). A slight downward change has been reported in the MMR, but it is too early to determine the impact of the village-based midwifery program.

- Bolivia, Egypt, Honduras, and Yunnan (China) are moving from situations in which the majority of women have been delivering at home with a relative or TBA (Model 1) to those in which they are delivering primarily with a skilled birth attendant in a facility (a mix of Models 3 and 4). Of these settings, Egypt, Honduras, and Yunnan have lowered their MMRs between 30 and 50 percent in the past decade. Bolivia's MMR has been reported only once during this period.

- Jamaica, where the majority of women deliver with a skilled attendant in a facility (Models 3 and 4), is trying to improve the quality of care and referral between facilities (improved Models 3 and 4); no change in the MMR has been reported.

- Zimbabwe, where the majority of women deliver in a facility with a skilled attendant (Model 3), has very unfortunately reported a large increase in the MMR between 1994 and 2000.

Methods

The country case studies were conducted using two primary methods: a retrospective case study approach, developed and used in Honduras, Yunnan (China), and Zimbabwe, and a research study approach involving the examination of data on maternal mortality and on specific interventions for Bolivia, Egypt, Indonesia, and Jamaica. Both methods relied on a mix of secondary and primary data sources, with the emphasis of the retrospective case study approach on the former and the research studies on the latter.

The retrospective case study approach attempted to collect data that spanned decades. The principal investigators developed a guide sheet of desirable data items based on the pooled experience from numerous country-specific assessments done in two international programs: the MotherCare Project of John Snow, Inc. (1989–2000), funded by the U.S. Agency for International Development (USAID), and The Maternal Health Programme of The London School of Hygiene and Tropical Medicine (1990–2001), funded by the U.K. Department for International Development. As the first case study emerged from Zimbabwe, more questions were added to the guide, and in China and Honduras, hypotheses were generated to direct the data collection.

Investigators obtained the information to answer the guide questions and test the hypotheses by reviewing the published literature, visiting key agencies in-country to obtain unpublished reports, and questioning key informants. Semistructured interviews with key informants, based on question guides, were conducted in Bolivia, China, Honduras, and Zimbabwe. Investigators chose key informants, who included officials and local leaders and health providers such as midwives and doctors, for their specialist knowledge of, or insights into, issues of relevance to the inquiry.

In the research studies (and in some of the retrospective case studies), other means augmented available reports and literature. In Bolivia, Honduras, Jamaica, and Yunnan (China), researchers undertook data collection efforts at health facilities, using clinic records and registers. Such collection depended on the scope and purposes of the investigation and the quality of the available data. In many settings, such as Egypt, health facility records are scantily kept and their quality is poor. Investigators also conducted focus groups with health providers, women, female patients, and TBAs in Honduras and Zimbabwe and, in Bolivia, exit interviews with women attending antenatal care. The Egypt, Honduras, Indonesia, and Jamaica studies capitalized on ongoing research studies. In Egypt and Honduras, for example, the reproductive age mortality surveys (RAMOS) of maternal mortality provided the basis for the case studies, whereas the Bolivia and Indonesia case studies depended on data collected during the MotherCare Project (1995–2000) (for example, pre- and postsurveys and clinic records).

Results

There are two types of results: one related to the methods used to collect the information and the other related to the content of the studies.

Methodological Results

The advantages and limitations of the case study methodology are best explored in the context of a conceptual framework, Determinants of Health Outcomes (figure 1.1) (Claeson and others 2001). While most useful in determining "successful" factors within current health system sectors and government policies and actions, the case study methodology leaves gaps in the information, especially from the past and the household and community levels. In particular, information on subjects best studied using qualitative methods proved difficult to locate and to compare over time. For example,

Figure 1.1 Determinants of Health Outcomes

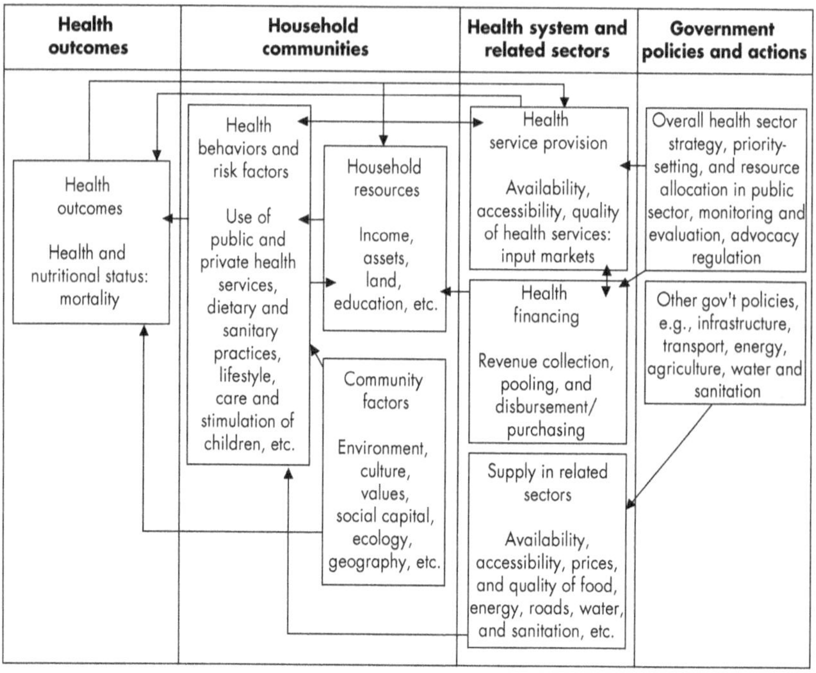

Health outcomes	Household communities	Health system and related sectors	Government policies and actions
Health outcomes Health and nutritional status: mortality	Health behaviors and risk factors Use of public and private health services, dietary and sanitary practices, lifestyle, care and stimulation of children, etc. Household resources Income, assets, land, education, etc. Community factors Environment, culture, values, social capital, ecology, geography, etc.	Health service provision Availability, accessibility, quality of health services: input markets Health financing Revenue collection, pooling, and disbursement/ purchasing Supply in related sectors Availability, accessibility, prices, and quality of food, energy, roads, water, and sanitation, etc.	Overall health sector strategy, priority-setting, and resource allocation in public sector, monitoring and evaluation, advocacy regulation Other gov't policies, e.g., infrastructure, transport, energy, agriculture, water and sanitation

Source: Claeson and others 2001.

data on how women perceive the quality of care and the value they place on using different services were not available. It was also difficult to establish whether past policies, plans, and strategies articulated by leaders had actually been implemented. For instance, community participation in providing and monitoring services, assumed to be important in present-day public health efforts, might be alluded to in plans but was not clear in practice. Similarly, data on the actual scope and content of supervision were rarely clear. Some of these data were collected for current programs, as in Bolivia, Honduras, and Zimbabwe, but represented only the present and only the site where they were obtained (that is, not the entire country).

Other missing data include the skill level of providers (especially to perform essential obstetric care) and the capability of facilities. Data on training curricula were usually available, but those on the performance of providers rarely so. Data on the actual functional capability and resources of different facilities, including those in the private sector, and their ability to refer and to manage complications were also unavailable. In fact, the terminology used to describe facilities was unclear; the same terms might describe completely different institutions. Data on met need, assessed by looking at complicated cases admitted to bEOC or cEOC, also could not be found. Good indicators for quantifying appropriate referrals were lacking, and hence such patterns remain unknown. Additionally, while current programs aim to increase general knowledge about danger signs in pregnancy, delivery, and postpartum, this was not discussed in the country settings we studied.

Finally, it was difficult to identify appropriate persons in-country to conduct the case studies: these individuals needed to understand the particularities of maternal health care issues while having a sufficient breadth of experience to tackle policy issues. They also needed the skills to relate interventions to quantitative population-based data on their coverage and impact.

Substantive Results

The main results were a series of seven case studies, a synopsis of which follows this summary chapter. These case studies have built on the delivery configurations derived from analysis of the historical case studies of rural China, Malaysia, and Sri Lanka (table 1.1). That analysis signaled possible factors leading to the countries' successes (Koblinsky, Campbell, and Heichelheim 1999). But whereas the prominent factors (shown in table 1.3) were found almost consistently in the three historical case studies, they are not in the new case studies. For example, in all the historical and present case studies, there is high availability of both skilled birth attendants and birthing facilities, but not all the present cases have strong policy guiding their programs, and only one holds its medical personnel accountable.

Table 1.3 Factors Associated with Reduced Maternal Mortality Ratio

FACTORS ASSOCIATED WITH REDUCED MMR < 100 PER 100,000 AND THEIR DEGREES OF IMPORTANCE	HISTORICAL ANALYSIS	CURRENT ANALYSIS
High availability of skilled birth attendants located near the home, especially where home births are traditional	+++	+++
High availability of birthing facilities	+++	+++
Free or reduced costs for services and transport to the services for clients	++	+
Strong government policy guiding the health program, usually including the maternal health programs	+++	+
Formalized referral links among facilities and the providers, including community providers such as TBAs	++	+
Providers accountable to the public for their performance	++	+

Note: MMR = maternal mortality ratio/100,000 live births. + indicates factor found in case studies, the number of +s indicating how often, with +++ being the highest.

Discussion

The case studies of the seven settings provide us with insights into programmatic elements associated with maternal mortality reduction. The methodology, historical case studies, is new and as such has both limitations and benefits. The major benefit is that we now know elements governments implemented through their programs to address maternal deaths. The discussion below elaborates on the methodology and these programmatic elements.

Methodological Limitations

Because we are deriving explanations with hindsight, the association of the successful factors with a reduction in MMR or even an increase in the use of services is merely ecological. None of the countries, except Jamaica, used experimental designs to implement interventions; randomized controlled designs would have provided more conclusive evidence of an effect. In addition, we rarely have enough disaggregated data to allow us to compare subregions and areas. The possibility that the countries we selected are unrepresentative could be a further limitation. The case studies were largely conducted in countries that measured and reported MMRs. This could lead to an overemphasis on the importance of measurement, or conversely the emphasis on reporting the MMR may be an important factor in stimulating action (Van Lerberghe and De Brouwere 2001).

We note that all the above factors could also limit prospective evaluations of maternal health care when nonexperimental designs are used and signal areas of research yet to be developed.

Factors for Success

The six factors of success listed in table 1.3 were not witnessed in each setting reviewed, but the effect of their implementation in specific settings is instructive and is discussed below.

Increased availability of a skilled birth attendant. A health worker with midwifery skills present at childbirth, supported by transport in case emergency referral is required, is perhaps the most critical intervention for making motherhood safer (Starrs 1997). A skilled birth attendant is defined as a health worker with midwifery skills providing care for normal deliveries and basic EOC. To be highly effective, the attendant needs to have an enabling environment that includes drugs, medical supplies, and a referral system with doctors providing emergency obstetric care (Graham, Bell, and Bullough 2001). This occurs most easily when birth takes place in a referral health facility (Model 4) but, as historical case studies show, can be achieved within Models 2 and 3 as well.

Increasing the use of a skilled birth attendant has become the major focus of international safe motherhood programming. However, major questions concerning the skilled birth attendant strategy include the following:

- At what population level should the skilled birth attendant be posted?
- What skills should the attendant have?
- Where should the attendant practice?

Table 1.4 Availability of Skilled Birth Attendants

IDEAL VS. COUNTRY	SKILLED BIRTH ATTENDANT PER NUMBER OF PEOPLE	CRUDE BIRTHRATE	POTENTIAL LIVE BIRTHS ATTENDED PER YEAR
Ideal (per ICM and FIGO)	1/5,000	40	200
Egypt	1 ob-gyn/3,500	28	100
Indonesia	1 village midwife/1,000	23	23
Malaysia	1/4,000	25–50	100–200
Zimbabwe	1 midwife (health center)/1,000	31	31

Note: FIGO = International Federation of Gynecologists and Obstetricians; ICM = International Confederation of Midwives.

Analysis of the case studies informs the first of the two questions.

The International Confederation of Midwives (ICM) and the International Federation of Gynecologists and Obstetricians (FIGO) propose one person with midwifery skills per population of 5,000 (WHO 1999). Assuming an annual crude birthrate (CBR) of 40 per 1,000 people, then a skilled birth attendant would manage approximately 200 births a year, presumably ensuring retention of his or her skills. In the 1960s and 1970s, when she was delivering the majority of babies in the home, the Malaysian midwife conducted 100 to 200 births annually (see Liljestrand and Pathmanathan 2002).

In many of the case study settings, the ratio of skilled birth attendant (typically a trained midwife but in Egypt also an obstetrician) to births is much higher than that recommended by the professional associations or experienced in Malaysia, while fertility is lower (table 1.4). Both Indonesia and Zimbabwe report one midwife per population of 1,000. Since Indonesia has only 23 births per 1,000 (CBS and others 1998), the Indonesian village-based midwife could on average provide care for 23 births per year if all pregnant women in her village sought her assistance for delivery. In the period 1992–97, however, only 31 percent of rural Indonesian women delivered with a skilled birth attendant, so village-based midwives may have delivered less than one birth per month (CBS and others 1998).

Zimbabwe's CBR was 31 births per population of 1,000 in the mid-1990s, so each midwife could potentially conduct 31 deliveries annually. In 1992–97, 61 percent of all births were assisted by a midwife and a further 12 percent by a doctor (73 percent total with a skilled birth attendant), and 72 percent of births occurred in health facilities. Zimbabwean midwives work in health centers and do not typically conduct home births. In such settings where women appear willing to use facilities for birthing, the skilled birth attendant can have a good clientele without visiting the households and can also provide such care in a team (which most providers seem to prefer over delivering women alone in the home).

In Egypt the estimate is one obstetrician per population of 3,500. With a CBR of 28 per 1,000, an obstetrician could conduct around 100 births annually, provided all women delivered with them. Estimates for 1995–2000 suggest that, in practice, doctors attend 54 percent of births, or 54 births a year on average per obstetrician. Many obstetricians work in individual-physician private clinics (one per population of 8,700–11,000), of which 69 percent provide delivery care with a reported average of 48 deliveries a year. Obstetricians have 2.1 jobs on average, and most also work for the Ministry of Health and Population (MOHP), where they conduct hospital births.

Based on the cadre and length of training, one would expect midwives in Indonesia and Zimbabwe to have a lower skill level than the obstetricians in Egypt. There are no national data on the actual skills of these providers, although small studies in Indonesia and Egypt indicate competency-based skills are considerably lower than might be expected for a given cadre. When the skilled birth attendant delivers 100–200 births a year (8–16 babies a month), he or she is likely to retain the skills needed to provide basic essential obstetric care. But when the attendant delivers fewer than 3 births a month (as in Indonesia and Zimbabwe), then specific skills requiring more practice, such as manual procedures for placental removal or breech presentation, may be lost over time.

The skill level of the attendant needed at the most peripheral setting also depends on the ready accessibility and acceptance of referral care. In Yunnan, China, where fertility is low and referral seems relatively available, the skills of the village doctor are aimed at normal delivery and at recognizing problems and stabilizing the patient, rather than at managing complications. There is one village doctor (upgraded barefoot doctor) per population of 1,000–1,500 in Yunnan, and while they can and do deliver normal births, they do not have a midwife's skill level. However, their referral support is relatively close and seemingly accessible to Chinese women.

In summary, the ideal population size served by a skilled birth attendant, the skills needed, and where the attendant provides care (for example, home, clinic, hospital) depend on a number of factors, such as the birthrate, female mobility and acceptance and use of a static birthing center, and the resources and commitment of the government to provide skilled maternal health care close to the community, including a referral system. Both the degree of urbanization and population density probably play important roles as well, since it is easier to place staff and facilities when populations are denser. Getting the right balance of skills, distance to women, and health system support for the skilled birth attendant begs for experimentation on the part of a government in places where women do not avail themselves of a skilled birth attendant. To date no published data on any such experiments have been found.

Increased availability of health facilities to provide skilled birthing care. WHO (1994) and UNICEF recommend one cEOC facility and four bEOC facilities for every 500,000 people (1 bEOC per 125,000). As with the skilled birth attendant, successful countries appear to go beyond this level of recommended availability. In two counties of Yunnan, China, for example, there is at least one cEOC facility for every 100,000 people and a bEOC facility (and sometimes a cEOC) for every 30,000. In Egypt, there is one hospital for every 32,000–42,000 (most of these are likely to provide at least bEOC, if not cEOC) and one private provider–led clinic offering delivery care (bEOC) per 13,000–16,000. Indonesia and Zimbabwe also have a bEOC facility for every 30,000. Our case studies also yielded other examples of bEOC facilities besides a government health center with beds: the dedicated birthing center and the private provider clinic or facility. The maternity waiting home also emerges as a strategy for increasing access to facility births for remote or dispersed populations.

The population base per facility is only one indicator of availability, however, and it can mask geographic features that hinder access, such as mountains and rivers. More precise indicators of availability are distance and time from a woman's home to facilities, as provided in the Service Availability Modules (SAM) used in conjunction with the demographic and health surveys (DHS), 1993–96, for Zimbabwe and Indonesia (Rose and others 2001). Similar data are available from an earlier period for rural women in Egypt (Sayed 1991).

At the time of the SAM, more than three-quarters of Zimbabwean married women ages 15–49 and 80 percent of those in Indonesia lived in rural areas. With a similar level of infrastructure, approximately 25 percent of rural Zimbabwean women and 38 percent of rural Indonesian women were within 5 kilometers of a facility with delivery care. Travel time to existing facilities with delivery care was less than an hour for 35 percent of Zimbabwean women and for 88 percent of Indonesian women. Median travel time for delivery care for women in Zimbabwe was 90 minutes, with about 70 percent walking, while it was 15 minutes in Indonesia, with 60 percent using motorized means. Yet availability of services is clearly not the full story: 61 percent of rural women in Zimbabwe used a health facility for birthing at the time of the survey, while only 8 percent of rural Indonesian women did, despite having greater availability of birth facilities in terms of distance and time from their homes. Other factors, such as the cost of services and cultural beliefs, continue to impede use (cost is discussed below).

In a few of the successful countries, two types of health facilities within the maternal health field have extended access beyond government clinics and hospitals—birthing homes or private provider clinics, and maternity waiting homes.

Birthing homes are typically community places where women can go to give birth with a skilled provider. Often built and maintained by community members, such homes draw skilled providers to the area. They have been used in Honduras (Danel 1999) and Cuba (Cardoso 1986) and are presently being tried in Guatemala (Bocaletti, Bratt, and DeLeon 1995). In Indonesia, village-based midwives may also have a delivery bed at their offices. The potential of birthing homes is great in not only increasing use of a skilled birth attendant but also acquainting the clinically skilled providers with the more cultural aspects of birthing by, for example, partnering them with community health workers, such as the TBAs. The 13 birthing homes built in the rural remote areas of Honduras where the MMR was highest in 1990 were providing care for approximately 4,000 of the 190,000 annual births in the country by 1997. Given the remoteness of such areas and the strong traditions of home delivery, it is possible that a majority of births in the birthing centers were complicated. By providing skilled attendants and enabling them to refer women for further care if necessary, it is estimated that 6 to 10 percent of expected maternal deaths (approximately 12 to 20 deaths) were avoided (Danel 1999).

In Egypt, a substantial number of births are conducted in private provider clinics. These are similar to government birthing homes in that they are largely dedicated to delivery care and are probably equipped to a bEOC level, but unlike government facilities, they are less likely to be placed in areas of greatest need.

Maternity waiting homes are typically built near hospitals; they are places women can go near the time of delivery that offer easy access for a facility delivery. Maternity waiting homes have successfully extended access to referral hospitals in Honduras, Zimbabwe, and other countries.

- In the remote rural areas with an MMR of higher than 300 in 1989, Honduras built five maternity waiting homes near level 1 hospitals. Women at extremes of age, having their first birth or fifth or more birth, or with underlying medical problems were referred to the waiting homes in anticipation of a possible poor outcome. TBAs and other community workers as well as nurses and doctors staffing health clinics were trained in this risk assessment and instructed where to send women. A 1999 study in six referral hospitals, conducted over a one-month period, found that hospitals with maternity waiting homes were significantly more likely than those without to have women referred to them and these women were more likely to be older and grand multiparous (see Honduras Case Study).

- Beginning in the early 1960s, Cuba established a network of hospital services for the entire population to increase the number of deliveries by skilled attendants. The government paid special attention to the rural areas where access and communications were extremely difficult. It enlarged existing hospitals and built new ones in rural areas. Maternity waiting homes were set up in the vicinity of the hospitals so that women from remote areas could be accommodated during their final weeks of pregnancy. The first maternity waiting homes were opened in 1962; by 1984, there were 85 homes, with 1,461 beds. As a result, the proportion of institutional deliveries increased from 63 percent in 1963 to 99 percent in 1984. Maternal mortality fell from 118 to 31 per 100,000 births during this time period (Cardoso 1986).

- Central Ethiopia's first maternity waiting home opened in 1976 to service the catchment population of the private Attat Hospital, forming part of the maternity services in the rural areas. The home was intended for pregnant women "at risk," the majority of whom had multiple risk factors. The positive impact of that home and others subsequently established was assessed in a study that found 13 maternal deaths among women admitted directly to the hospital versus the absence of deaths and of ruptured uteri among the women using the maternity waiting home. The stillbirth rate was 10 times higher among the direct hospital admissions than among the women admitted from the homes. The study's authors concluded that maternity waiting homes are critical for women who have to travel long distances, have only poor transport, and where obstetric disasters are frequent (Poovan, Kifle, and Kwast 1990).

- Maternity waiting homes also reduced adverse perinatal outcomes in Zimbabwe. The perinatal mortality rate was 32 per 1,000 live births for those who came directly from their own homes to the hospital during labor versus 19 per 1,000 among women who stayed in the maternity waiting home, an almost 50 percent reduction (Chandramohan, Cutts, and Millard 1995). Similar strategies have been used for dispersed and remote populations in Alaska, Australia, the Kentucky Frontier, Mongolia, and Scotland.

High use of facilities for birthing and the level of maternal mortality are inversely related. Unfortunately, available data do not distinguish between cEOC and bEOC centers, and whether the emergency obstetric capability drives the mortality reduction remains unclear. Uptake of services is the primary outcome of high availability of facilities. When use of such services does not take place despite high availability, as in Indonesia, the existence of other barriers to access, such as cost or culture, needs to be considered.

Facilities such as birthing homes and private clinics may provide a means for relieving the overflow of maternity patients without complications in hospitals and, together with maternity waiting homes, for accessing referral care needed by patients with complications in rural settings. Particularly in the Latin American and African context, in which home birth by skilled attendants is not a programmatic strategy, such facilities may prove an important means of providing for professional care at birth and a primary means for facilitating appropriate care for those with greater clinical needs.

Service costs appropriate for the setting. While Malaysia, Sri Lanka, and initially rural China reduced their MMRs over decades by providing free or highly accessible health care (or both) to all, many countries now charge fees for health services. Reports of fees decreasing use of health facilities for births began to appear in the 1990s; their impact on use of emergency obstetric care is increasingly recognized (Ekwempu and others 1990). To address this problem, Bolivia implemented an insurance strategy that diminishes or eliminates user fees. Indonesia extended the limit for its social safety net upward to ensure that women can use health facilities when needed. To what extent have these strategies been successful?

Bolivia's National Maternal and Child Health Insurance (MCHI) Program went into effect in mid-1996, covering prenatal, labor and delivery, and postpartum and newborn care, including cesarean section and management of all obstetric and newborn complications. In late 1998 the government augmented the MCHI with the Basic Health Insurance (BHI) to explicitly cover complications at any phase of the maternity period, including postabortion care and transfers of emergency patients. The BHI also provides an incentive for priority interventions in facilities. Between 1994 and 1998, women in rural areas increased their use of a skilled birth attendant from 26 to 34 percent. Women in the poorest quintile showed the greatest increase in use of skilled care for births—from approximately 11 to 20 percent—and in use of public health facilities for those births, from 7 to 14 percent (Gwatkin and others 2000). Overall, facility deliveries (in urban and rural areas) rose from 42 to 56 percent. There was no increase reported in cesarean sections for rural women; the rate remained at approximately 6 percent throughout this period (INE and MI 1994, 1998). Because the poorest quintile has such low levels of skilled birthing care, however, the bulk of insurance funds actually cover the costs of those who are better off, most of whom already use skilled birthing care.

In 1997, an economic crisis swept Indonesia, affecting the gains the country had made in safe motherhood since initiating its village-based midwife strategy in the early 1990s. The government had ensured the availability of a skilled birth attendant in every village but appeared not to give equal priority to hospital care. The cost of a cesarean section in South Kalimantan, a province on the island of Borneo, was reported at US$240 in 1996, a fifth of the average national gross domestic product (GDP) per capita at the time. No change in this pricing was seen, even when inflation hit. In response to inflation, Indonesia increased the income level considered eligible for the social safety net that covered hospital care; hospitalized women relying on the safety net increased from 1.5 to 11.4 percent between 1997 and 1999. However, those receiving cesarean sections actually decreased—from 1.7 to 1.4 percent ($p = 0.005$), as did those admitted to the hospital with an obstetric complication—from 1.1 to 0.7 percent ($p = 0.001$) (see Indonesia Case Study).

The high cost of delivery services to families appears to be a major factor hindering use. Yet in both the Bolivian and Indonesian contexts, the cost to families does not seem to be the only factor determining uptake. A large portion of the Bolivian poor remain outside services even with free care, and poor Indonesian women who could qualify for the social safety net do not access facilities even when complications occur. Whether the lack of use in both countries is due to lack of knowledge of the free service (its existence, where it can be found, or how it can be obtained), to cultural differences in birthing, or to other barriers remains unknown. But reduction of costs alone does not seem to redress the lack of facility use by those most in need.

Strong policy guidance for delivery care. Government policy in historical cases, such as those of Sri Lanka in the 1940s and China and Malaysia in the 1950s, was focused not on maternal mortality reduction, but on the equity of health care for all. This translated not only into the presence of frontline providers close to women's homes, where most births occurred, but also into a support infrastructure for these providers that included the capability to refer and manage complications. Services were free to the consumer, thus eliminating one financial barrier. In Malaysia and Sri Lanka, transport to the referral facilities was also provided, eliminating a second financial barrier.

In 1957 newly independent Malaysia determined that access to health care for all was an important step for the government. The country planned to achieve equitable health care by posting one well-trained midwife for every 2,000 people, with the skills to provide prenatal, delivery, and postpartum care in a woman's home, as well as family planning, child health care, and first aid for the entire population. The midwife could provide oxytocics and other drugs; would have access to a public health nurse for antibiotics, suturing, or intravenous fluids; and could call for transport to a hospital for further care. Sri Lanka had a similar approach to providing health care for all but had begun its midwifery program several decades before Malaysia.

China ensured access to health care for all through a different level of cadre. With the formation of the People's Republic of China in 1949, a community worker named a barefoot doctor was selected from each commune to provide first aid. Trained briefly and often informally, the barefoot doctors could aid in uncomplicated birthing if requested but did not have much instruction beyond the level of a trained TBA. However, an essential element we postulate as linked to reducing China's maternal mortality was that the barefoot doctors could refer patients to higher-level care with surgical capability. Hence barefoot doctors needed to be able to recognize complications but did not have to manage them.

In these success stories, all three countries decided to promote facility-based births after they could already show that a good proportion of women were in the government's home-based professional health care system. Starting from this position of strength (that is, with the health system already in charge of home-based birth), the shift to facility-based birthing took place in approximately a decade—the strategies to shift care following governmental policy guidance.

While China, Malaysia, and Sri Lanka took decades to reduce their maternal mortality from levels of 600 and above, Honduras reduced its MMR from 182 in 1990 to 108 in 1997, a 41 percent decline in just seven years (Danel 1999; see Honduras Case Study). A major difference between the historical success stories and that of Honduras is that the latter's policy explicitly targeted maternal mortality reduction, rather than equity of health care for all.

Shocked by a 1990 RAMOS study reporting a higher than desired MMR, the Honduran Ministry of Health (MOH) strategically planned to reduce maternal mortality through multiple approaches, including improvements in infrastructure, personnel levels, and strategies to increase use and improve quality of care. Resources for infrastructure and donor support were directed to areas with the highest MMRs (greater than 300), identified through a survey. Six years later, the results in rural areas showed that use of a skilled birth attendant had increased by a third (from 24 to 32 percent between 1990–91 and 1996), but that use of cesarean sections had increased only slightly. A greater percentage of maternal deaths now occurred in facilities, suggesting a shift of complicated cases to hospitals, although still not in time for the women to be saved.

Over the short term, infrastructure improvements included new community health clinics, maternity waiting homes, birthing homes, and dozens of rural health clinics and several rural hospitals in the areas of need. More health staff was hired, trained, and deployed; TBAs were "integrated" into the health care system; norms were published; and TBAs and other health personnel were oriented to focus on women with "reproductive risk." Simultaneously, a general policy aimed at decentralizing the health system reportedly enhanced community involvement, stimulating local communities to use resources to resolve their issues and to build and maintain birthing centers and maternity waiting homes.

Honduras's efforts to target specific geographic areas, motivated by the MMR from the surveillance study, appear to have paid off. Knowledge of the MMR has also proved a powerful stimulus to policy formation in a number of other countries, including Bolivia, Indonesia, and Jamaica. If, as in Honduras, these policies are followed by the targeting of resources to needy areas, it is anticipated that other successes in maternal mortality reduction could be achieved relatively rapidly.

A functioning referral system, beginning with providers at the community level. "Use of referral" is the end step of a multifaceted effort. At the family level, referral begins with the recognition that the pregnant woman has a medical problem or a risky status that makes her or her baby vulnerable to a poor pregnancy outcome. To reach a decision on whether to use a bEOC or cEOC facility, the family may bring together people outside the immediate family whose opinion is highly regarded—a traditional birth attendant, a local healer, the mother-in-law, or another relative. Decisionmaking typically revolves around an assessment of the level of danger or risk and the perceived effectiveness of health providers or referral sites in managing it. Decisionmaking also takes into consideration the logistical problems, such as the costs (monetary, time, other household needs), distance, and transport. In many countries, it is the husband or another male family member who makes the final decision about using such services.

In Model 1, recognition of complications and effective household decisionmaking on seeking care in case of emergency may be essential; unfortunately, baseline knowledge of the signs of the five major obstetric complications is typically low. Creating awareness of danger signs among TBAs and among pregnant women has not proved easy, and the messages are complex. For example, even after a three-year period of disseminating information through radio talk shows and communications materials based on qualitative research, knowledge of the danger signs of hemorrhage increased only approximately 20 percent among women (MotherCare Matters 2000). More recently, information, education, and communications (IEC) campaigns and community mobilization efforts have focused on not only improving the awareness of danger signs and where to go for help, but also helping make preparations for possible costs and transport.

Within the health system, in Models 2 and 3, referral, too, is multifaceted. Providers at the different levels of care need protocols that guide them in determining at what point in the course of a complication, or at what level of risk, they should refer the woman. These protocols also need to address how to prepare the woman for referral, how to communicate with the referral level, how to ensure transport between the levels, and how to counsel the family and woman to promote adherence to referral. When women are accustomed to giving birth outside health facilities, a bridge between the family, community, and referral facility may be required. That role can be played by a frontline provider such as a midwife, as in Malaysia, or it can be carried out by a community worker trained to recognize, refer, and coordinate with the health services, as in China and Honduras. Local organizations outside the health system, such as nongovernmental organizations (NGOs) or women's groups, may also be effective in these liaison tasks, as has been reported from Kenya (Macintyre and Hotchkiss 1999) and Guatemala (Bailey, Bocaletti, and Holland 2000).

Honduras was able to ensure appropriate referrals through a "risk focus" strategy implemented in the early 1990s. This has two prongs: ensuring that women who developed obstetric emergencies are referred to the hospital, and identifying women at higher risk for complications or poor pregnancy outcomes and encouraging them to deliver in a health facility. The training of clinical staff and community health workers (including TBAs) focused on danger signs in childbirth (such as bleeding, hypertension, labor longer than 8 hours for multiparas or 10 hours for primiparas, premature rupture of membranes, fever, retained placenta, and malpresentation) and on risks (such as extreme age, first birth, more than four births, and underlying medical problems). Women and families were made aware of the danger signs and risks during prenatal care. Levels of prenatal care use increased from 73 percent in 1987–91 to 83 percent in 1995–2000, with an even greater increase in the rural areas (from 67 to 81 percent). Norms published in 1995 emphasized identification and referral to the hospital of high-risk women and those with obstetric emergencies.

Through this risk focus, and by increasing the availability of appropriate staff and birthing facilities (as described above), it is likely that more Honduran women who needed referral care were delivered at an appropriate level (see Honduras Case Study for details). A one-month study of all deliveries in six referral-level hospitals showed that 48 percent of the 59 referrals during labor and delivery had a documented complication, compared with 20 percent among the 1,106 deliveries not referred. The figures were 17 percent versus 9 percent for a cesarean section, 10 percent versus 2 percent for a stillbirth, and 17 percent versus 8 percent for newborns with a problem after delivery.

TBAs contributed 42 percent of these referred women, and their referrals were usually appropriate. This suggests that TBAs are referring women with obstetric complications for hospital delivery and that they feel comfortable with, and have confidence in, the health services to respond appropriately and well. TBAs often accompany the women to the hospital. Similar results for TBA referral were seen in a project in Forteleza, in northeastern Brazil, in the early 1980s (Janowitz and others 1988; Koblinsky, Campbell, and Heichelheim 1999).

The study in Honduras also showed that significantly more women over age 34 or with more than four births were among those referred. The data suggest that the maternity waiting homes increased the likelihood that high-risk women would have a hospital birth.

The risk approach that underlies this Honduran strategy was promoted by WHO in the early 1980s as a means of selecting pregnant women most in need of referral and management. It was based on both risks (for example, age, parity, previous pregnancy and medical history, socioeconomic status) and danger signs of medical problems, and relied on a scoring system to determine the overall level of risk for the woman and where she should deliver. The risk approach (particularly its risk prediction aspects based on age parity and socioeconomic status) fell into disfavor among researchers as studies showed it was neither sensitive nor specific enough on a population level to accurately predict which women would suffer obstetric complications or maternal death (Akalin and Maine 1996; Chandramohan, Cutts, and Chandra 1994; Tsu 1994). It had a high rate of false positives, and in settings such as Guatemala, where, for example, the MOH has stated it could manage only 20 percent of deliveries in health facilities, it could easily overwhelm the system (Koblinsky and others 2000). However, where it is the norm for women to deliver at home alone or with a community worker such as a TBA or with a relative—as was the case in Honduras, Malaysia, and northeastern Brazil in the early 1980s—knowing that certain characteristics make a woman more vulnerable to a bad outcome can be a trigger for referral among lay workers as well as lower-level health staff. Their efforts have been deemed appropriate by hospital staff, particularly when the aim is to increase all facility births, as in Honduras and Malaysia.

Even where women use health services, effective risk assessment that focuses on diagnosing health problems can improve referrals and care. In Jamaica, where eclampsia is the biggest killer of pregnant women, midwives were trained specifically in blood pressure diagnosis and urine testing to identify women with hypertension or preeclampsia during antenatal care. They were supported by obstetricians hired to attend such women in high-risk clinics. Even so, it was found that both pregnant women and community workers needed to know the signs of hypertension to catch women when they needed care. Women were provided with small picture cards depicting such characteristics as a swollen face or swollen hands, and community health aides were trained to recognize these signs and to alert women to the fact that uncomfortable walking could also mean a problem. These interventions proved pivotal: before the intervention pregnant women with hypertensive disorders occupied about six beds per day, whereas after the intervention, fewer than three beds per day were so occupied and the numbers of eclampsia admissions were dramatically reduced. No such changes occurred in the control areas (see the Jamaica Case Study).

Accountability for providers' performance. Since the 1992 World Summit for Children, China has given high public visibility to maternal mortality reduction at the national level. On an annual basis, for example, governors must publicly provide information on the MMR of their provinces. They in turn hold their provincial-, county-, and township-level officials accountable for the local MMRs. Strategies for achieving a lowered ratio are developed at the provincial level. This system was felt to have played a major role in maintaining the low MMR in the Chinese countryside following the move from a free-service policy to a fee-for-service one in the early 1980s.

For example, beginning about 1980, Yunnan Province (home to approximately 42 million people in 1999) adopted multiple strategies for decreasing maternal mortality, including a stated policy to increase hospital deliveries; high availability of facilities able to provide essential obstetric care (as detailed above); a frontline provider, the village doctor, able to identify problems and refer women in need, located close to women (at a population level of 1,000–1,500); a referral system among facilities and providers linked by performance-based contracts and periodic meetings for supervision; demand creation through an insurance scheme to decrease the costs of prenatal and postpartum care; and a pilot study on an insurance scheme to decrease delivery costs.

When it moved to a fee-for-service system in the early 1980s, China anticipated that doctors would provide only curative care because they could earn more for it than for preventive care. In Yunnan, however, officials determined that provision of the preventive services, prenatal and postpartum care, was important and therefore incorporated use of these services, as well as use of facilities for deliveries, into the performance contracts. Through various indicators that form a necessary part of the service contracts used by health facilities in commissioning lower-level facilities, officials monitor how well each level is doing in achieving the expected outcomes of the provincial strategies. An example of a performance indicator is the rate of systematic management of pregnant women (SMPW). The SMPW includes providing every woman with a systematic management booklet (educational booklet on the content and necessity of care throughout the maternity period), at least five prenatal checks, a minimum of three postnatal visits in her home (the first within 24 hours of delivery), and the new methods for home delivery if she has one (clean perineum, clean birth attendant hands, and clean umbilical cord). The SMPW, the percent use of hospital delivery, and the decrease in the MMR together compose the systematic management rate (SMR). Scores for performance of each level of care within a county are based on these quantitative indicators. They are, in turn, used in determining subsidies for facilities and even continuation of employment for lower-level providers (village doctors). While the subsidies linked with the SMR are modest, ranking based on the score is considered an overall appraisal of the maternal and child health (MCH) services and is closely tied to promotion of managers.

Malaysia also used indicators and targets of facility performance to determine progress. The country's quality assurance approach, aimed at ensuring the adequacy of hospital care, went into effect in the mid-1980s. Obstetricians determined that the percent of hospitalized women with puerperal sepsis and the percent with eclampsia were two indicators that spoke to the quality of care. Hospitals with and without specialists are compared twice yearly in accordance with these indicators and the targets set by the specialists. Outliers are obliged to investigate the reasons for poor performance. As in China, those responsible for health care must publicly state, on an annual or a semiannual basis, whether they have achieved their targets and their plans for improvements (Koblinsky, Campbell, and Heichelheim 1999).

Whereas the indicators of progress in Yunnan, China, are aimed primarily at use of specific services, those of Malaysia are aimed at *quality of care*. But both sets of indicators have proved powerful because they quantify results linked with specific strategies and interventions, and in themselves have driven action.

Challenges of the Future

In addition to the six programmatic factors elaborated above, these case studies provide themes and developments that are only partly understood at present but may prove important in the future. These include the role of political and economic crises, as seen in the cases of Indonesia and Zimbabwe, and their impact on the relative costs and access to essential care; the contribution of culture in societies, such as Indonesia, that appear to be resistant to facility births; the future role of decentralization and planning and management capacity at lower levels and how this will pan out for maternity care, as illustrated in Honduras; the large role of the private sector, as seen in Egypt, and the difficulties in regulating quality; and finally the rising toll of pregnancy-related mortality seen in settings with large HIV/AIDS problems, as in Zimbabwe.

A late 1980s community-based study in a rural and an urban area of Zimbabwe provided MMRs of less than 200 and 100, respectively. However, DHS data for 1988–92 and 1995–99 confirm an upward trend in pregnancy-related mortality, a trend reported from neighboring Malawi as well. AIDS-related conditions and malaria are two culprits taking their toll on pregnant women as indirect causes of maternal death. They are also weakening the health service systems that have been in place. Special efforts to focus on these indirect causes of maternal death where they are prevalent must receive a higher priority.

Conclusions

The stimulus for this study was the question, Can current program strategies reduce maternal mortality more quickly than the historically successful countries of Malaysia and Sri Lanka? The answer appears to be no. The decline in the MMRs by 30–50 percent to approximately 100 or less in Egypt, Honduras, and Yunnan (China) took 7–10 years in the 1990s. Malaysia and Sri Lanka also needed 7–10 years to achieve a similar MMR level, in the mid-1960s to mid-1970s.

There are caveats to this answer, however. First, the historical successes were tracked back in time to when they had MMRs of 500 or more, while the case studies reported here have an MMR of less than 200 at the earliest time of our data collection. Prior data for the latter are generally unavailable or unreliable. When a country has achieved an MMR of 200, it appears there is already momentum toward reducing the MMR. Typically, a third or more of women are already using skilled birth attendance. Second, the historical successes have multiple MMR data points, mostly drawn from adequate government sources, whereas the data points for the MMRs in these case studies are generally only two. Perhaps their MMRs were lower in a shorter period of time, but no information is available.

Like Malaysia and Sri Lanka, the countries reported in this volume also use multifaceted approaches to lower their MMRs, with high availability of skilled birth attendants and supportive facilities where women can go for management of complications being two very prominent features. Targeting resources to increase such availability in geographic areas with high MMRs, as well as intervening with a mechanism that triggers awareness and use of care specifically in cases of high risk or obstetric complications, has proved a successful strategy in Honduras. Reaching an MMR of approximately 100 with only 54 percent of women being aided by a skilled birth attendant means that women with complications are getting the care they need. The momentum to use these services increases perhaps as such practices become a social norm.

While the six programmatic factors outlined in this paper seem to underlie the success in these country case studies, the limitations of the retrospective case study methodology mentioned earlier also limit our understanding of the priority of these factors. Only the health system and policy factors were captured by the methodologies used and are hence highlighted. Household- and community-level factors, so difficult to capture, particularly over time, are likely to play a role in increasing the use of a skilled birth attendant and reducing the MMR, but which factors, and the relative importance of all factors, remain unknown. Given this and other unknowns now playing a role in present day programming for Safe Motherhood, such as health care reform and infectious diseases (HIV/AIDS), the need to document successes as well as failures will remain vital to continued progress.

References

Akalin, M. Z., and D. Maine. 1996. "Strategy of Risk Approach in Antenatal Care: Evaluation of the Referral Compliance." *Social Science and Medicine* 41(4):595–96.

Bailey, P. E., E. Bocaletti, and H. B. Holland. 2000. "Using Hospital Obstetric Data to Monitor Utilization and Referral Patterns in Guatemala." Manuscript in preparation for Family Health International, Research Triangle Park, N.C.

Bobadilla, J. L., F. S. Reyes, and S. Karchmer. 1996. "Magnitude and Causes of Maternal Mortality in the Federal District, 1988–89 (in Spanish). *Gac Med Mex* 132(1):5–16.

Bocaletti, Elizabeth, J. Bratt, and H. DeLeon. 1995. *Comparative Costs of Normal Delivery at the Hospital and Community Maternity Center in Guatemala.* MotherCare/Guatemala, Guatemala City.

Cardoso, U. 1986. "Giving Birth Is Safer Now." *World Health Forum* 7:348–52.

CBS (Central Bureau of Statistics) (Indonesia), NFPCB (State Ministry of Population/National Family Planning Coordinating Board), MOH (Ministry of Health), and MI (Macro International Inc.). 1995. *Indonesia Demographic and Health Survey, 1994*. Calverton, Md.: CBS and MI.

———. 1998. *Indonesia Demographic and Health Survey, 1997*. Calverton, Md.: CBS and MI.

CSO (Central Statistical Office) (Zimbabwe) and MI (Macro International Inc.). 1995. *Zimbabwe Demographic and Health Survey, 1994*. Calverton, Md.: CSO and MI.

———. *Zimbabwe Demographic and Health Survey, 1999*. Calverton, Md.: CSO and MI.

Chandramohan, Daniel, F. Cutts, and R. Chandra. 1994. "Effects of a Maternity Waiting Home on Adverse Maternal Outcomes and the Validity of Antenatal Risk Screening. *International Journal of Gynecology and Obstetrics* 46(3):279–84.

Chandramohan, Daniel, F. Cutts, and P. Millard. 1995. "The Effect of Stay in a Maternity Waiting Home on Perinatal Mortality in Zimbabwe." *Journal of Tropical Medicine and Hygiene* 98:261–67.

Claeson, Mariam, C. C. Griffin, T. A. Johnston, M. McLachlan, A. L. B. Soucat, A. Wagstaff, and A. S. Yazbeck. 2001. "Poverty-Reduction and the Health Sector." In *The Poverty Reduction Strategy Sourcebook*. Washington, D.C.: World Bank.

Danel, Isabella. 1999. *Maternal Mortality Reduction, Honduras, 1990–1997: A Case Study*. World Bank, Latin America and Caribbean Region, Washington, D.C.

Ekwenpu, C. C., D. Maine, M. B. Olorukoba, E. S. Essien, and M. N. Kisseka. 1990. "Structural Adjustment and Health in Africa. *Lancet* 336(8706):56–57.

Graham, W. J., J. S. Bell, and C. H. W. Bullough. 2001. "Can Skilled Attendance at Delivery Reduce Maternal Mortality in Developing Countries?" In Vincent DeBrouwere and W. Van Lerberghe, eds., "Safe Motherhood Strategies: A Review of the Evidence." *Studies in Health Services Organisation & Policy* 17: 97–130.

Gwatkin, D. R., S. Rutstein, K. Johnson, R. P. Pande, and A. Wagstaff. 2000. "Socio-Economic Differences in Health, Nutrition and Population." Paper. World Bank, HNP/Poverty Thematic Group, Washington, D.C.

Institute of Health Sciences. 2001. *Maternal Mortality Reduction in Tonghai and Huaning Counties, Yunnan, China: A Case Study, 1981–1999.* Kunming, Yunnan.

INE (Instituto Nacional de Estadistica) (Bolivia) and MI (Macro International Inc.). 1994. *Bolivia Encuesta Nacional de Demografia y Salud, 1994.* Calverton, Md.: CBS and MI.

———. 1998. *Bolivia Encuesta Nacional de Demografia y Salud, 1998.* Calverton, Md.: CBS and MI.

Janowitz, Barbara, P. E. Bailey PE, R. C. Dominik, and L. Araujo. 1988. "TBAs in Rural Northeast Brazil: Referral Patterns and Perinatal Mortality." *Health Policy and Planning* 3(1):48–58.

Keeling, J. W., A. M. McCaw-Binns, D. E. Ashley, and J. Golding. 1991. "Maternal Mortality in Jamaica: Health Care Provision and Causes of Death." *International Journal of Gynecology and Obstetrics* 35:19–27.

Koblinsky, M. A., O. Campbell, and J. Heichelheim. 1999. "Organizing Delivery Care: What Works for Safe Motherhood?" *WHO Bulletin* 77(5):399–406.

Koblinsky, M. A., C. Conroy, N. Kureshy, M. E. Stanton, and S. Jessop. 2000. *Issues in Programming for Safe Motherhood.* Washington, D.C.: MotherCare/JSI.

Liljestrand, Jerker, and I. Pathmanathan, eds. 2002. *Investing Effectively in Maternal Health: Malaysia and Sri Lanka.* Washington, D.C.: World Bank.

MacIntyre, Kate, and D. R. Hotchkiss. 1999. "Referral Revisited: Community Financing Schemes and Emergency Transport in Rural Africa." *Social Science and Medicine* 49(11):1473–87.

MOH (Ministry of Health) (Egypt), Child Survival Project, in cooperation with USAID (U.S. Agency for International Development). 1994. *National Maternity Mortality Study (NMMS), 1992–1993.* Cairo, Egypt.

———. 2001. *National Maternity Mortality Study (NMMS), 2000.* Cairo, Egypt.

MotherCare Matters. 2000. *Behavioral Dimensions of Maternal Health and Survival.* Washington, D.C.: MotherCare/JSI.

Murray, S. F., S. Davies, R. K. Phiri, and Y. Ahmed. 2001. "Tools for Monitoring the Effectiveness of District Maternity Referral Systems." *Health Policy and Planning* 16(4):353–61.

Poovan, Pamela, F. Kifle, and B. Kwast. 1990. "A Maternity Waiting Home Reduces Obstetric Catastrophes." *World Health Forum* 11:440–45.

Rose, Amanda, N. Abderrahim, C. Stanton, and D. Helsel. 2001. *Maternity Care: A Comparative Report on the Availability and Use of Maternity Services. Data from the Demographic and Health Surveys Women's Module & Services Availability Module 1993–1996*. Measure Evaluation Technical Report Series No. 9. Chapel Hill: Carolina Population Center, University of North Carolina.

Sayed, H. A. A. 1991. *Egypt Service Availability Survey 1989: Availability and Accessibility of Family Planning and Health Services in Rural Egypt*. Columbia, Md.: Cairo Demographic Centre and Demographic and Health Surveys. Macro International Inc.

Starrs, Ann. 1997. *The Safe Motherhood Action Agenda: Priorities for the Next Decade*. New York: Inter-Agency Group for Safe Motherhood and Family Care International.

Stephenson, Patricia, M. Wagner, M. Badea, and F. Serbanescu. 1992. "Commentary: The Public Health Consequences of Restricted Induced Abortion—Lessons from Romania." *American Journal of Public Health* 82 (10):1328–31.

Tsu, V. D. 1994. "Antenatal Screening: Its Use in Assessing Obstetric Risk Factors in Zimbabwe." *Journal of Epidemiological and Community Health* 48(3):297–305.

Van Lerberghe, Wim, and V. De Brouwere. 2001. "Of Blind Alleys and Things That Have Worked: History's Lessons on Reducing Maternal Mortality." *Studies in Health Services Organization and Policy* 17:207–28.

WHO (World Health Organization). 1994. *Indicators to Monitor Maternal Health Goals. Report of a Technical Working Group. Geneva, 8–12 November, 1993*. Geneva: World Health Organization, Maternal Health and Safe Motherhood Programme. XX(32745.2).

———. 1999. "Skilled Care during Childbirth." Draft Report. Geneva.

WHO, UNICEF (United Nations Children's Fund), and UNFPA (United Nations Population Fund). 2001. *Maternal Mortality in 1995: Estimates Developed by WHO, UNICEF, UNFPA*. Geneva: WHO.

PART 1

Case Studies

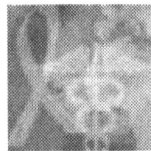

CHAPTER 2

Yunnan, China, 1980–1999
Institute for Health Science

China has reported a large decline in the maternal mortality ratio over three decades, from approximately 1,500 per 100,000 live births in 1950 to 100–200 in rural areas in 1980. Even with replacement of free services, through the cooperative medical system/insurance, with fee for service around 1978, the MMR has continued to slowly decline, registering 74 in rural China in 1998 (Ministry of Public Health, or MOPH). Although family planning does not contribute to a reduction in the MMR, China's successful program, advocated since the 1970s, has undoubtedly contributed to a decrease in the numbers of maternal deaths by reducing the total fertility rate from 5.81 in 1970 to below 2 in 1998 (figure 2.1).

Yunnan, one of China's poorest provinces, with an average gross national product (GNP) per capita of US$536 in 1999, reported an MMR of 101 in 1998, a drop from 149 in 1989. Home to 42 million people in 1999, Yunnan has an ethnic population of more than 10 million, one of only three provinces (and autonomous areas) with such a high ethnic population. Family planning has also been instrumental in Yunnan, where the TFR dropped from 5.25 in the 1970s to 2.20 in 1998.

In a study of Tonghai and Huaning, two agricultural Yunnan counties with differing socioeconomic status, the MMR in the better-off Tonghai stayed relatively low over the 19-year period from 1981 through 1999, averaging 52, while in Huaning, the MMR averaged about 84. Socioeconomically, Huaning is about average for

Figure 2.1 China: Maternal Mortality Ratio and Total Fertility Rate, 1950–96

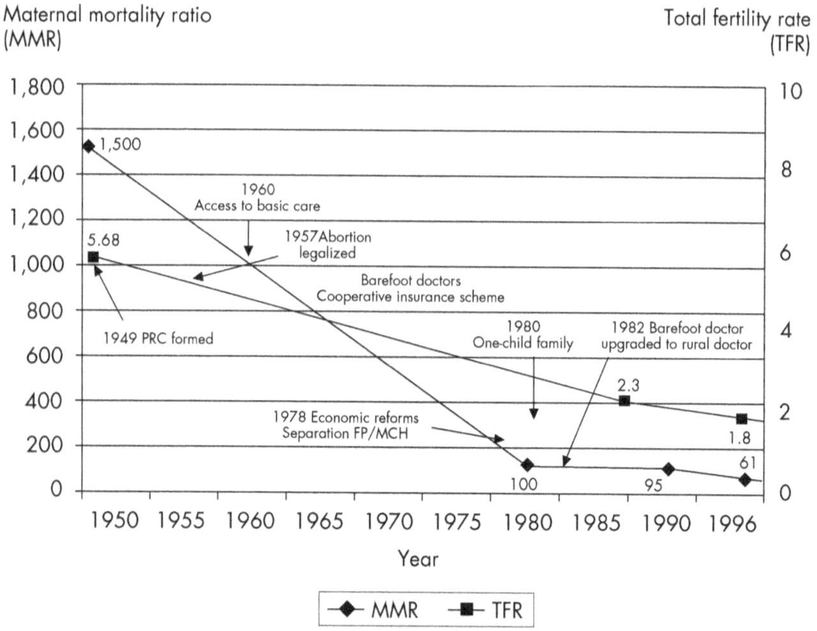

Maternal mortality ratio (MMR) / Total fertility rate (TFR)

Key events annotated on the figure:
- 1949 PRC formed
- 1957 Abortion legalized
- 1960 Access to basic care
- Barefoot doctors / Cooperative insurance scheme
- 1978 Economic reforms / Separation FP/MCH
- 1980 One-child family
- 1982 Barefoot doctor upgraded to rural doctor

Data points: MMR 1,500 (1950); TFR 5.68 (1950); MMR 100, TFR 2.3 (1980); MMR 95 (1985); MMR 61, TFR 1.8 (1996)

Source: Koblinsky, Campbell, and Heichelheim 1999.

Yunnan's 128 counties, with a 1999 per capita income of US$271; Tonghai is above average, with a 1999 per capita income of US$700. The populations of these two counties are small, however (260,000 in Tonghai and 195,000 in Huaning, in 1999), and annual births average around 3,500 and 2,700, respectively. Family planning use in 1999 in Tonghai was 86 percent and in Huaning, 88 percent, with resulting TFRs of 2.1 and 2.16, respectively.

In Tonghai in 1990, use of the hospital for delivery was already high, at about 70 percent; by 1999, it had risen to 92 percent. Women and families in this county largely use the county MCH station or county hospital for maternity care, both cEOC hospitals. For the less well-off county, Huaning, hospital deliveries were around 49 percent in 1990; they rose to 62 percent over the next nine years.

Here women largely use the township health center (THC) and village clinics for maternal care, both of them bEOC-type facilities, the former staffed with doctors (figure 2.2; table 2.1). Huaning is more geographically dispersed than Tonghai, making transport more difficult. Use of prenatal checks and postnatal visits is high in both counties, around 87 percent for either type of visit in Huaning and 96 to 97 percent in Tonghai. For women with high-risk pregnancies in both counties, use of prenatal and postnatal care has been 100 percent since 1996. High risk is defined by 10 conditions (including pregnancy-induced hypertension, small pelvis, abnormal fetal position, antepartum hemorrhage, twins, preterm labor, postterm preg-

Figure 2.2 Huaning and Tonghai Counties, Yunnan: Hospital Delivery Rates, 1990–99

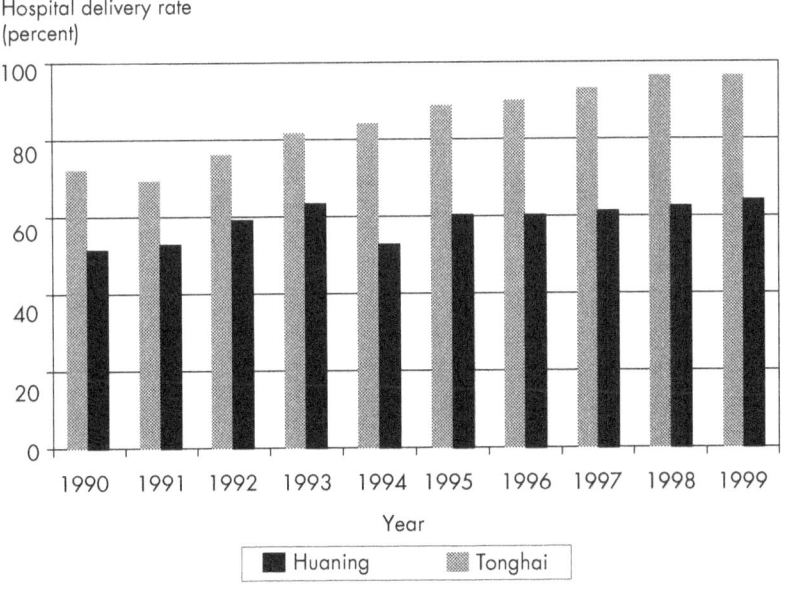

Source: County MCH Station, MIS, Huaning and Tonghai Counties, 1990–99, as reported in Institute for Health Science 2001.

Table 2.1 Huaning and Tonghai Counties, Yunnan: Maternity-Related Statistics, 1999

CATEGORIES	HUANING	TONGHAI
GDP (per capita in US$)	$272	$700
MMR[a] (average 1980–99)	84	52
CPR[b] (%)	88	86
Hospital delivery[a] (%)	62	92
Prenatal care[a] (%)	87	96
Postnatal care[a] (%)	87	97

Note: CPR = contraceptive prevalence rate.
a. County Statistical Yearbook, Huaning and Tonghai Counties.
b. County MCH Station, MIS, Huaning and Tonghai Counties, as reported in Institute for Health Science 2001.

nancy, other complications, or history of abnormal delivery or hydantidiform mole).

Strong Policy Guides the Way

Paving the way for such outcomes, China promulgated policies and laws promoting increased coverage for maternal and child health and for health education for at least 85 percent of pregnant women by 2000, with use of the modern delivery method for 95 percent of births with village doctors. This modern delivery method, used by village doctors, must include sterilization of the perineal region, the birth attendant's hands, and the umbilical cord. In 1991 the government stressed that the MMR would be halved by 2000 by increasing the delivery rate in hospitals for rural women. National and provincial regulations determined the MCH institutes' responsibilities, the quality of care standards, the equipment needed for family delivery by TBAs, personnel allowances, and medical aid for the poor.

Referral Links

A three-tiered health network provides maternal and childcare and forms the basis for referral (figure 2.3). At the village level lies the village clinic (VC), staffed by at least one village doctor (about half the village doctors in Tonghai and Huaning are female). Prior to 1978, this level was the production unit, and the village doctors were called barefoot doctors. The village clinics provide prenatal care checks and postpartum home visits, refer high-risk women to hospitals for delivery, and monitor the work of TBAs in their areas. The town level (previously the commune level) has a township health center (THC) or township hospital, with beds for delivery and a staff of professional doctors (about half the THCs and township hospitals are cEOC facilities, the others are bEOC). At the county level can be found not only a county hospital but also the county MCH station, which is responsible for MCH care for the population, as well as for training, supervising, and monitoring the township and village MCH personnel, including the village doctors and TBAs. The county-level facilities have at least one operating room, a laboratory with the capacity to bank blood, and a pharmacy (cEOC facil-

Figure 2.3 Yunnan: Three-Tiered Maternal and Child Health Care Network

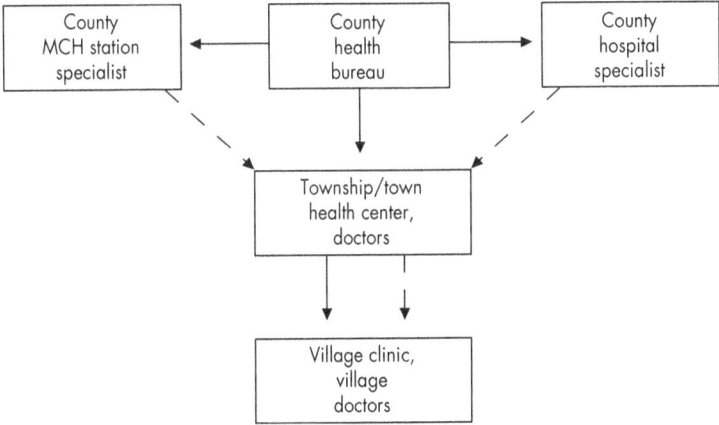

Note: A solid arrow signifies an administrative relationship, a broken arrow a professional one.
Source: Institute for Health Science 2001.

Table 2.2 Huaning and Tonghai Counties, Yunnan: Health Care Infrastructure, 1999

HEALTH CARE INFRASTRUCTURE	HUANING			TONGHAI		
	NUMBER	PER POP. (LEVEL POP. # = 195,000)	PER LIVE BIRTH LB (# = 2,683)	NUMBER	PER POP. (LEVEL POP. # = 260,000)	PER LIVE BIRTH LB (# = 3,496)
County hospitals	2	97,500	1,342	2	130,000	1,748
THCs	5[b]	39,000	537	8[a]	32,500	437
Village clinics	76	2,566	35	44	5,909	79
Village doctors	207	942	13	153	1,699	23
TBAs	115	1,726	24	42	6,190	83

Note: TBA = traditional birth attendant; THC = township health center.
a. 4 of 8 THCs are comprehensive hospitals.
b. 2 of 5 THCs are comprehensive hospitals.
Source: County MCH Station, MIS, Huaning and Tonghai Counties, as reported in Institute for Health Science 2001.

ities). In both counties, the level of potential contact with a part of this system is high. In Huaning, for example, there is one VC for every 35 live births and one THC for every 536; in Tonghai these ratios are one VC for every 79 and one THC for every 437 (table 2.2).

In the 1970s barefoot doctors taught themselves or received brief, irregular training from county and village health institutions. The institutions' topics included attending clean delivery and identification of risk factors and complications prior to, and during, delivery. Since 1982 government regulations have required those barefoot doctors wishing to be village doctors (VDs) to take an exam on these topics; if they pass, they earn a VD certificate. If they do not pass, they remain TBAs. The upgraded "village doctors" (or certified barefoot doctors) received a few months of on-site training. More recently, a new cadre of "modern village doctors" has received regular training of approximately three years, generally conducted by the county or prefecture health institutions, during which the doctors gain a general knowledge of obstetrics and gynecology and more information on risk factors and identification of complications. Continuing education for all village doctors is provided at monthly meetings. The community worker to population ratio is staggering: with more than 31,000 village doctors and 23,000 trained TBAs, Yunnan averages one village doctor per 1,400 people and one TBA per population of 2,000. In Huaning, there is one village doctor for every 13 live births, and in Tonghai, the ratio is one for every 23.

The links between the levels of care form the routine referral system whereby a woman experiencing a complication may move from the village clinic to the THC then to the county MCH station or hospital. In 1990 Tonghai formed the Emergency Referring System for Pregnant Women (ERS). The eight ERS strategies included establishing a county guiding group for coordination; ensuring functioning telephones at all levels; equipping emergency facilities, including vehicles; improving providers' skills by protocol; enhancing the three tiers; establishing a supervision and evaluation system; and bringing the ERS management into the target-oriented system. Standards for referral include referring when the placenta has not appeared within 30 minutes after the birth or referring any emergency within 30 minutes to a higher-level service. The ERS is credited with saving many lives, its survival rate for the emergency cases averaging 96 percent between 1990 and 1999.

Monthly meetings offer another means of integrating the providers at different levels of care: each lower-level meeting is organized by the immediate higher-level institution for discussions of the routine statistical report, problems and their resolution, exchanges of experience, training, and plans for future work. The information flow follows the referral system, with the data ultimately being sent to the county MCH stations and the analysis being fed back. Village doctors initiate the information collection and provide a monthly report based on four reports: births, deaths, the systematic management booklet for pregnancy, and a similar booklet for child management. The county stations forward the monthly, semiannual, and annual statistical reports to the prefecture MCH stations; the reports then go to the provincial level and finally to the MCH Department of the MOPH. Information is highly valued and statistical training is provided for personnel at the different levels of care.

Program Implementation: Action with Accountability

While China promulgates policies at the national level, strategies to ensure their implementation are determined at the provincial level or below. In Yunnan, the management system allows for higher-level institutions to contract with lower MCH sectors for specific tasks on which they are scored using quantitative indicators (such as the systematic management rate, or SMR). The lower sector is held accountable for these tasks over a specific time period, with financial subsidies and promotion of managers closely related to the scores achieved. Examples of indicators include the percentage of women delivered in the hospital, the decrease in the MMR, and the systematic management of pregnant women (SMPW). The SMPW includes providing every woman with a systematic management booklet, at least five prenatal care checks, a minimum of three postnatal visits in her home (the first within 24 hours of delivery), and the new methods for home delivery.

Despite the modesty of the subsidies linked with the SMR, the rank of scores is considered an overall appraisal of the MCH services and is closely related to the promotion of managers. At the community level, evaluation of the village doctors and health workers is related not only to subsidies but also to their employment: if they do not satisfy their supervisors, they may lose their jobs. Because the program stresses preventive reproductive health services, evaluations linked with employment status ensure that such preventive care is actually provided, although higher fees are obtainable for providing more curative care. For example, since the SMPW was implemented in Tonghai in 1985 and in Huaning in 1986, informants from the county MCH station and the County Health Bureau believe that village doctors and TBAs are screening a larger number of women for risk and referring them to the hospital for delivery. In 1995 in Huaning, 11 percent of pregnant women were determined to be high risk; among the 286 high-risk women who delivered, 242 were in the hospital (85 percent). This same system of scoring works not only below the county level but also above it (that is, at the prefecture level).

Ensuring Financial Accessibility

Even though the SMPW strategy ensures that all clients will receive basic MCH care, county-level managers found it difficult to raise the SMR further despite improvement in the availability and quality of services. To improve service utilization, many other schemes have been tried: one that has been popular in Yunnan is the MCH Prepay Scheme, piloted in a demonstration county before becoming available throughout the province. In general, the scheme asks new couples in the rural areas to pay a modest fee at the time of marriage registration to cover future prenatal (five checks) and postnatal care (three visits) and several child health exams. If certain complications associated with delivery or diseases of the child arise, the family can claim compensation. The cost of the scheme may vary by site, but in Huaning, the total fee was nearly equal to what it would cost a woman for one prenatal or postpartum visit to the county hospital alone! The fees are not considered too much for households to pay; however, poor women do enjoy free MCH services outside the scheme. Research suggests that those who joined the scheme would seek MCH services more actively.

The prepayment scheme does not include delivery charges, however. Delivery charges vary from county to county; in Nanhua County, Yunnan, in 1998–99, they cost US$124.41 at the county hospital, US$75.25 for the county MCH station, and US$29.97 for the THC. Indirect costs for transport, food, and other items increase the charges by a third to nearly one-half as much as the delivery fees, with lower indirect expenses at the THC level. A new program, titled Medicaid for Poor and High Risk Pregnant Women, will soon be implemented and tested in Tonghai and Huaning Counties to cover hospital delivery for these women.

Summary

Following the transition to a fee-for-service system, the MMR has been maintained at a low level (MMR less than 100) in two rural districts of Yunnan through implementation of an accountability system that motivates providers, especially village doctors, to ensure comprehensive MCH care (preventive and curative) to families. To lessen the financial barriers to access, specific insurance schemes provide good coverage of prenatal and postpartum care, and experiments for coverage of delivery are now being piloted. The village doctors provide prenatal and postpartum care through home visits and identify high-risk pregnancies for delivery in higher-level facilities, although the quality of their skills is unknown. The infrastructure to population ratio supports a very high level of contact with the population (one VD per population of 1,000–1,500; one THC per 35,000; one cEOC per 130,000).

Very strong political will and visibility around maternal mortality (one of three main indicators reviewed annually and publicly at the national level) and around pregnancy guide this system of care. This national focus on maternal mortality has ensured that information on pregnancies, where women deliver, and death is followed carefully throughout the system.

References

Institute for Health Science. 2001. *Maternal Mortality Reduction in Tonghai and Huaning Counties, Yunnan, China: A Case Study, 1981–1999*. Kunming, China. Report prepared for JSI Research and Training Institute.

Koblinsky, M. A., O. Campbell, and J. Heichelheim. 1999. "Organizing Delivery Care: What Works for Safe Motherhood?" *WHO Bulletin* 77(5):399–406.

CHAPTER 3

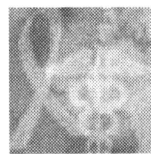

Honduras, 1990–1997
Isabella Danel with Ada Rivera

In 1997 the MMR in Honduras was measured at 108 per 100,000 live births, making it a country with "low" maternal mortality (Melendez, Ochoa, and Villanueva 1999). Only seven years before, in 1990, it had been as high as 182 per 100,000 (Castellano, Ochoa, and David 1990). This case study examines some of the strategies adopted by Honduras to reduce its maternal deaths.

Attendance at Birth

By 1997 Honduras had moved to having skilled attendance for the majority of its estimated 191,000 annual births. According to the national epidemiology and family health survey (ENESF), during the five-year period 1992–96, approximately 54 percent of women giving birth had a skilled attendant, while 39 percent were attended at home by a traditional birth attendant and 7 percent received no assistance whatsoever (ENESF 1997). Nearly all births with skilled attendance took place in hospitals and were attended by physicians. Less than 1 percent of births occurred at home with a skilled attendant. Approximately 2 percent occurred in birthing centers.

All hospitals in Honduras are cEOC facilities, staffed by specialists from obstetrics and gynecology; all have at least one operating room and the capacity to bank blood and provide anesthesia. First-level MOH referral hospitals (*area* hospitals, n = 17 for the country) can refer patients to secondary (*regional*, n = 6) or tertiary (*national*, n = 2) hospitals. Secondary and tertiary hospitals are located in larger urban towns (population greater than 100,000 population) and the two metropolitan areas (nearly 1 million each). They therefore function not only as referral centers for women outside the immediate area, but also as first-level referral hospitals for women living in those cities. These eight hospitals attend approximately 53 percent of the facility-based births in Honduras—or 29 percent of all births (Danel 2000).

Approximately 8 percent of all births occur at one of two Social Security Institute hospitals (many salaried workers receive social security health insurance), and 6 percent occur in private hospitals or clinics.

In 1998 approximately 2 percent of births took place in birthing centers (Honduran MOH 1999). These centers provide basic essential obstetric care, generally have transport available in case of emergencies, and are staffed by a professional nurse with special training in obstetrics. They are less expensive to maintain than hospitals and bring skilled attendance closer to pregnant women living in harder to reach areas. The centers are generally constructed and maintained with the support of the community in which they are located. The MOH opened the first center in 1985; by 1993, six had been inaugurated. This strategy has become increasingly popular and has been adopted by a wide range of communities. By 1997 there were 13 birthing centers—by the end of 1999, 23. Each attends anywhere from 100 to 1,000 births a year (Honduran MOH 1999). Birthing centers offer a skilled attendance alternative to secondary and tertiary hospitals in larger towns and cities—one that also reduces hospital overcrowding and thus potentially allows the hospitals to provide better care to women with obstetric complications who really need it.

Honduras is currently expanding its birthing centers and is shifting toward a combination of Models 3 and 4. However, for the period 1988–97, Honduras made a transition from Model 1 to Model 4, that is, from a majority of home births with TBAs to a majority of births with skilled attendants, mostly in cEOC hospitals. What caused this transition?

Policy Leading to Increased Availability of Services

The 1990 RAMOS study that focused on maternal mortality helped galvanize the efforts behind these changes: knowledge that the MMR was 182 gave the Ministry of Health a "rude awakening" (Danel 2000). Targeting regions of the country with the highest MMRs (regions 2, 5, and 6), the government, with donor assistance, built seven new rural area hospitals and, with community input, five maternity waiting homes attached to rural hospitals as well as eight new birthing centers. The number of urban medical health centers (CESAMO) and rural health centers (CESAR) also increased. While these health centers do not provide delivery care, they do offer prenatal care and referrals for hospital delivery for high-risk women.

Throughout the country, an increase in the number of health personnel, especially auxiliary nurses, accompanied the rise in facilities. More training was offered. The training of the clinical staff, along with community health workers (including the TBAs), focused on recognizing risks in pregnancy (extremes of age, first birth, more than four previous births, underlying medical problems) and danger signs in childbirth (including bleeding, hypertension, labor longer than 8 hours for multiparas and 10 hours for primiparas, premature rupture of membranes, fever, retained placenta, and malpresentation). Norms for the integrated care of women were published in 1995; they emphasized the identification and referral to hospitals of high-risk women and those with obstetric emergencies.

Referrals

In considering the interplay between the use of formal birthing services and the decrease in the MMR, two questions emerge: What factors contributed to the slow but steady increase in demand for birthing services from 46 percent in 1987–91 (ENESF 1992) to the point where slightly more than half of women now have skilled attendance during delivery (54 percent)? And given that 54 percent is still a relatively low level of skilled attendance, how has the MMR declined to 108? Many countries with much higher levels of skilled attendance have similar MMRs, and countries with similar levels of skilled attendance have higher MMRs. There is no one answer to the second question. But one of the more intriguing strategies implemented in Honduras was a "risk focus" with an emphasis on improving referrals.

The risk focus was an MOH strategy developed during the early 1990s to improve maternal health. Officials implemented a two-pronged approach: ensure that women who develop obstetric emergencies are referred to the hospital and identify women at higher risk for complications and encourage them to deliver in a health facility. The MOH published and disseminated two training manuals focusing on this approach: one for TBAs and one for clinical staff, particularly staff providing prenatal care. The MOH later published a manual on management of obstetric emergencies in the hospital. The publication of these manuals was followed by training aimed at ensuring that TBAs and other health personnel were aware of the new recommendations and would implement them.

Improving Referrals for Obstetric Emergencies

In 1990 TBAs attended approximately 40 percent of births, particularly in rural areas where maternal mortality was high. Health personnel from the MOH and from NGOs carried out TBA training using the new manual. An attempt was made to train all TBAs, and community focus groups suggest that somewhere between 70 and 80 percent of TBAs have participated in the training. It included the recognition of certain danger signs during labor and delivery (including those listed above), and the immediate referral of women with those signs to the hospital. Health staff followed up this initial training in many, though not all, health areas; the staff held monthly meetings with TBAs to discuss problems they encountered and to reinforce what had been learned. It is difficult to assess the extent to which TBAs have incorporated the recommendations into their practices. However, it is clear that in some rural areas the relationship between TBAs and the formal health sector has improved.

Focus groups with TBAs and others with women from the local communities suggest that there have been changes in behavior secondary to the training. TBAs could articulate some of the danger signs and said they were referring more women during labor and delivery. They were also aware that some traditional practices were discouraged because they could be dangerous. Women in the local communities acknowledged the risk of going to an untrained TBA.

In a study of deliveries during a one-month period at six first-level referral hospitals (Rivera 2001), 5 percent of the deliveries (59 of 1,165) were among women who had planned to deliver at home but developed some type of problem during labor or postpartum. Two percent of women (25) stated that a TBA had convinced them to come to the hospital. TBAs accompanied 10 women, whom they had referred, to the hospital. TBAs also accompanied 4 other women after either the woman or her family made the decision to seek care at the hospital.

The women referred by TBAs in this small study were appropriately referred. Of the 25 women referred by TBAs during labor and delivery, 14 (56 percent) had a complication documented on the medical record compared with 20 percent of women not referred. Complications included seven women with prolonged labor, three with hemorrhage, three with premature rupture of membranes, and one with fetal distress. Most of the women with no documentation of a complication on the chart were referred for prolonged labor or malpresentation. Five of the women referred by TBAs (20 percent) had a cesarean section (compared with 9 percent not referred), and seven of the women, or 28 percent, had a poor perinatal outcome—either mortality or morbidity—compared with 8 percent of those not referred (see table 3.1).

Women and their families also seem to understand danger signs, as 29 of the 59 women who came to the hospital during their labor or postpartum stated that they or their families made the decision to do so. The study did not assess how much the TBA influenced this decision. When all the referrals during labor and delivery are grouped together (n = 59), 48 percent of women have a documented complication (compared with 20 percent of women not referred in

Table 3.1 Honduras: Referrals to Hospitals before and during Delivery, by Different Factors, 2000

FACTOR	REFERRAL BEFORE DELIVERY		REFERRAL DURING DELIVERY		
			YES—TYPE OF ATTENDANT		
	YES	NO	TBA	ANY	NO
Number of births	254	911	25	59	1,106
Risk status (%)					
High risk (age <18 or > 34, births > 4)	40	37	48	56	37
Very high risk (age > 34, births > 4)	31a	20	36	39	22
Complication on medical record (%)	33a	18	56a	48a	20
Cesarean section (%)	19a	6	20	17	9
Perinatal mortality or morbidity (%)	10	8	28a	27a	8

a. $p < 0.05$.

labor or delivery), 17 percent had a cesarean section (compared with 9 percent), and 27 percent had a perinatal mortality or morbidity (compared with 8 percent). Perinatal complications include stillbirths (10 percent of all women referred versus 2 percent not referred) and neonatal morbidity (17 percent versus 6 percent).

This information suggests that TBAs are referring women with obstetric complications for hospital delivery, that their referrals are usually appropriate, and that they often accompany women to the hospital. Since no baseline values exist, it is not possible to assess quantitatively whether there has been an increase in referrals following TBA training. Furthermore, the information suggests that women and their families are themselves aware of danger signs and may sometimes be the primary decisionmakers on whether to go to the hospital.

Birthing centers (with their bEOC) are an approach to increasing skilled attendance that should improve the timeliness of referrals for obstetric emergencies. As mentioned above, the first birthing center was constructed in 1985; by 1997 approximately 4,000 births (2 percent of all births) were occurring in these centers (Honduran MOH

1999). The numbers may be relatively small, but it should be noted that many of these birthing centers lie in remote areas with high maternal mortality, areas where women are disinclined to go to a hospital. If it is assumed that the MMR in these areas for women delivering at home is between 300 and 500, it can be estimated that, in 1997, between 12 and 20 maternal deaths were avoided because of birthing centers.

Referrals of High-Risk Women for Hospital Delivery (the Risk Approach)

The second part of the referral strategy was to increase the likelihood that women at higher risk for complications were referred for a hospital delivery. This was a pragmatic response to the fact that most rural women did not want to deliver in a hospital. If all women could not be immediately persuaded to go to a hospital, perhaps at least some of those at greater risk might be. Two easily recognizable risk factors are extremes of maternal age (particularly older maternal age) and grand multiparity; in every country of the world, MMRs are higher among these women. Health officials also consider women with serious problems in previous pregnancies to be high risk. Finally, women who develop problems during their pregnancy (such as hypertension, anemia, bleeding, and premature rupture of membranes) are also referred to the hospital for delivery.

This particular strategy was carried out in several ways. Health personnel were trained in this concept and referred high-risk women identified during prenatal care. TBAs and other community health workers were also trained to recognize high-risk women and encourage them to deliver in the hospital.

Because it sometimes proved difficult for women living in remote rural areas to go to the hospital when labor began, maternity waiting homes were constructed, with community assistance, alongside several of the hospitals. The relationship between hospitals and maternity waiting homes is loose, and clear direction for the homes' operation and supervision is not available. In some homes hospital physicians visit pregnant women on a daily basis, but not in all. No one has incorporated the records from the maternity waiting home into the health information system. The communities maintain the maternity waiting homes, whose purpose is to allow rural women to await the onset of labor in a place close to the hospital. In practice, many women (often older) who have had multiple births also come to the maternity waiting homes because they wanted a tubal ligation postpartum. A small registration fee is charged by some of the waiting homes (LP5–10).

During a one-month period in six first-level referral hospitals in Honduras, 24 percent of all women who gave birth received referrals prior to delivery and 84 percent of all women referred had written referrals: 60 percent were referred by a health center, 21 percent by a private doctor, 8 percent by a TBA, 7 percent by another hospital, and 5 percent by a birthing center. Women referred for a hospital delivery were significantly more likely to be older and to have had more than four births previously (grand multiparity). This suggests that the risk approach is indeed functioning. Hospitals with a maternity home were significantly more likely to have women referred to them, and these women were more likely to be older and grand multiparous (see table 3.2). This suggests that maternity waiting homes increase the likelihood that high-risk women will have a hospital birth. Hospitals in regions with a large decline in maternal mortality were also more likely to have women referred to them, and these women were older and grand multiparous (table 3.2).

The high level of referrals is associated with an increase in prenatal care. Nationally, prenatal care coverage increased from 73 percent in the five-year period prior to 1991 to 83 percent in the five-year period prior to 2000. However, the increase proved much greater in rural areas (from 67 to 81 percent) than in metropolitan (from 80 to 88 percent) or other urban areas (from 81 to 83 percent). There is now very little difference among rural, metropolitan, and other urban areas with respect to prenatal care coverage—81, 88, and 83 percent, respectively (ENESF 1997, 2002).

Table 3.2 Honduras: Referrals to Hospitals vis-à-vis Maternity Waiting Homes and Decrease in Maternal Mortality, by Different Factors, 2000

FACTOR	HOSPITAL WITH MATERNITY WAITING HOME		HOSPITAL IN REGION WITH >40% DECREASE IN MATERNAL MORTALITY	
	YES	NO	YES	NO
Number of births	667	498	734	431
Risk status (%)				
High risk (age < 18 or > 34, births > 4)	40	36	37	38
Very high risk (age > 34, births > 4)	25a	20	27a	20
Women referred to hospital at any time (%)	31a	14	40a	13
Complication on medical record (%)	22	22	24	21
Cesarean section (%)	9	9	12a	8
Perinatal mortality or morbidity (%)	11a	6	11a	7

a. $p < 0.05$.

Links between the Health System and TBAs

Incentives for the TBAs to participate in trainings and to interact with health staff include a medical bag, supplies and their refills, and an identity card that potentially gives them a better reception during referrals at hospitals, according to focus group discussions with TBAs. However, TBAs complained that these expectations were often not met and that the cost of transportation to the monthly meetings was often not reimbursed.

Their training in danger signs has resulted in knowledge of such complications as breech, obstructed labor, placenta previa, and retained placenta, and of risk signs of edema, migraine, and short-birth interval. The TBAs also mentioned that they "no longer make mothers push, as the women would get tired" (Rivera 2001), and that they fear delivering a woman known to be at high risk due to "legal problems" (Rivera 2001), loss of reputation, and loss of their ability to refer to health establishments. Hence, perhaps out of improved knowledge of complications, fear of repercussions, or both, TBAs are reportedly making more referrals. This is corroborated by the fact that 8 percent of all hospital referrals were by TBAs, and 42 percent of those referred during labor and delivery.

The training on pregnancy risk factors and danger signs of delivery has reached beyond the TBAs to include voluntary health workers, weight monitors, and voluntary malaria assistants. Asked about risks and signs, these cadres described them in a manner similar to that of the TBAs. One of the findings of the focus groups, not surprisingly, was that the relationship between community level workers and hospital staff depends on the attitude of the person in charge.

Women's Perspective on Use of Services

In focus groups, women listed several factors that prevent them from giving birth in hospitals. They include feelings of embarrassment and fear of the hospital's negative image, the lack of money to pay for transportation and hospital services, bad roads, lack of transport or fear of crime at night, no one to care for their children, and short duration of labor. Facilitators for accessing birth at a hospital include referral by a TBA or health personnel, concerns for safety, complications, and the ability to meet their need for surgical sterilization.

Has Quality Improved?

In focus groups, providers mentioned specific barriers to the provision of obstetric care in emergency situations: blood is not always available and the law does not allow hospitals to buy it; skilled providers are not always available at night, on weekends, and during holidays; ambulances for hospitals are lacking or nonfunctioning; equipment needed for deliveries is missing, including even delivery beds in some hospitals; patients have been rejected from hospitals by the guards; and there is poor sanitation and hygienic care.

Providers also felt that hospital budgets, purchase of supplies and equipment, and selection of management of the hospitals have been too centralized; with decentralization of the budgets for hospitals in 2002, they believe they will be able to manage a better quality of care.

Multifaceted Approach

This study observed an association between hospitals with high levels of referrals, particularly referrals of high-risk women, and greater declines in maternal mortality. The impact of this strategy was noted to be greater in hospitals in regions where maternal mortality was very high (greater than 300). However, one hospital in a department with a large decline in maternal mortality (55 percent) did not have a high level of referrals. This department (Yoro) began with a lower level of maternal mortality of 185 (Melendez, Ochoa, and Villanueva 1999). While the MOH explicitly focused its resources and intervened more in areas where maternal mortality was higher, and this seems to have paid off (with generally greater declines where mortality was higher initially), these same interventions may not be as successful or as necessary in areas where mortality is lower. Ideally, interventions need to be adapted to the problems encountered in each region. Why the MMR declined in Yoro is not clear, but it is not due to higher levels of referrals. The Hondurans seem to have been particularly successful at promoting a multifaceted approach to maternal mortality reduction (Danel 2000).

Conclusion

Between 1990 and 1997 Honduras moved from a Model 1 to a Model 4 country. However, the 40 percent decline in maternal mortality in that time period was achieved by certain modifications to Model 4. In particular, the focus on high-mortality areas, as well as on improving referrals of obstetric emergencies and high-risk women, seems to have paid off with a much steeper decline than might otherwise be predicted by an increase in skilled attendance from 46 to 54 percent. Finally, Honduras is also moving away from the more expensive Model 4 and since 1992 has been directing resources toward bEOC facilities staffed by professional and auxiliary nurses trained in obstetrics rather than toward a further increase in hospital capacity.

References

Castellano, Marel de Jesus, Jose C. Ochoa, and Vincent David. 1990. *Mortalidad de mujeres en edad reproductiva y mortalidad materna* (Women's Reproductive Age Mortality and Maternal Mortality). Honduran Ministry of Health. Honduras.

Danel, Isabella. 2000. "Maternal Mortality Reduction, Honduras, 1990–1997: A Case Study Carried Out for the World Bank." Background Paper. World Bank, Washington, D.C.

ENESF. 1992. *Encuesta Nacional de Epidemiología y Salud Familiar, 1990-91*. Honduras.

———. 1997. *Encuesta Nacional de Epidemiología y Salud Familiar, 1996*. Honduras.

———. 2002. *Encuesta Nacional de Epidemiología y Salud Familiar, 2001: Informe Resumido*. Honduras.

Honduran MOH (Ministry of Health). 1999. *Resumen de la encuesta nacional de las clínicas materno infantiles* (Summary of the National Survey of Birthing Centers). Maternal and Child Health Department, Women's Health Unit.

Melendez, J. H., J. C. Ochoa, and Y. Villanueva. 1999. *Investigacion sobre mortalidad materna y de mujeres en edad reproductiva en Honduras* (Investigation of Maternal Mortality and Women's Reproductive Age Mortality in Honduras). Honduras.

Rivera, Ada, 2001. "Evaluation of Community Participation in Maternal Health and in the Referral Process for Childbirth in Hospitals." Background Paper. World Bank, Washington, D.C.

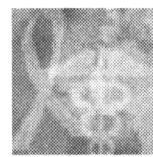

CHAPTER 4

Zimbabwe, 1980–2000

Shinga Feresu with Margaret Nyandoro and Leonard Mumbwanda

Zimbabwe is a relatively sparsely populated country (its population numbered approximately 12 million in 1997), with only a third of its inhabitants living in the urban areas. People in the rural areas are primarily farmers, either commercial or communal. Following independence in 1980, the country's new government developed a set of guiding principles for improving the lives of its people. One was the belief that everyone should be literate, and by 1992, the country had made great strides toward this goal, with 90 percent of men and 75 percent of women considered literate. Another guiding principle was based on the idea of health as a basic human right, with health care available, accessible, affordable, and acceptable to all regardless of race, ethnicity, creed, or social status. To address this principle, facilities were built in every district, health care staff were increased and trained, and roads and communications were ensured for all health facilities. One result of these actions was a drop in maternal mortality during the 1980s.

But Zimbabwe's story of maternal mortality has taken a detour on its road to success. In 1989–90 a community-based study in urban Harare and a rural area in Masvingo reported MMRs of 85 and 168, respectively, per 100,000 live births (Mbizvo and others 1994). Hospital and clinic data record a ratio of 100 per 100,000 live births in 1989, rising to 145 in 1997 (Feresu, Nyandoro, and Mumbwanda 2000) (figure 4.1). The Zimbabwe demographic and health surveys (ZDHS) show a far grimmer picture, with the MMR rising from 283 in 1994 to 695 in 1999, more than doubling the ratio (CSO and

MI 1995, 2000). The 1992 census gave an MMR of 395, confirming the higher level of maternal mortality. The proportion of all female deaths that are maternal has decreased, however, from 15 percent reported in data pre-1995 to about 10 percent in the 1999 ZDHS, meaning nonmaternal mortality is rising even more rapidly than overall mortality or maternal mortality. Infant and child mortality as well as the crude death rate (CDR) is also on the rise, as shown in table 4.1.

Yet pregnant women are for the most part delivering in a Model 3 or 4 setting: 72 percent of births were in health facilities in 1999,

Figure 4.1 Zimbabwe: Maternal Mortality Trends, 1988–99

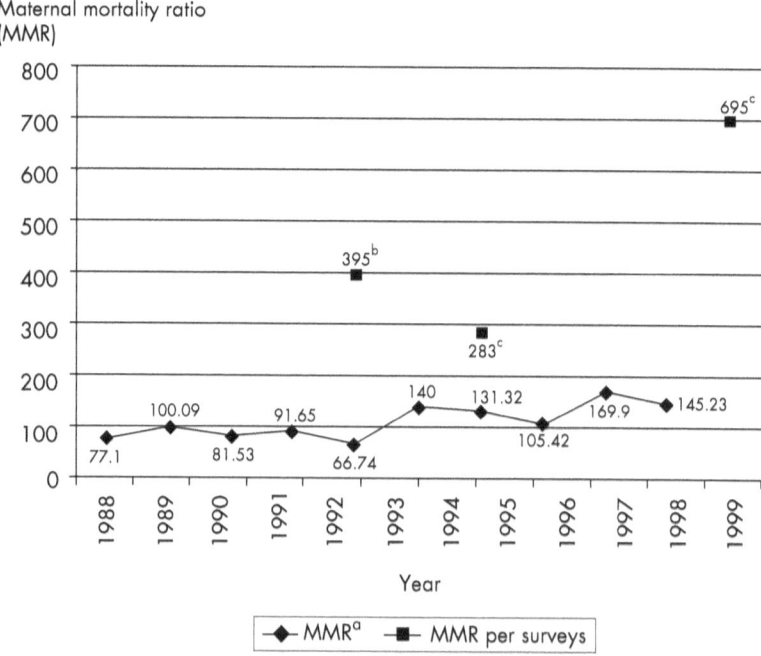

a. MMR = maternal mortality ratio/100,000 live births reported from government tally sheets, as reported in Feresu, Nyandoro, and Mumbwanda 2000.
b. Census 1992 as reported in Feresu, Nyandoro, and Mumbwanda 2000.
c. CSO and MI 1995, 2000.

Table 4.1 Zimbabwe: Select Demographic Indicators, 1962–97

INDICATOR	1962 CENSUS	1982 CENSUS	1992 CENSUS	1997 ICDS
Total population (million)	3.9	7.6	10.4	11.8
Crude birthrate (CBR)	48.0	44	43.5	34.7
Total fertility rate (TFR)	7.8	6.2	5.9	4.3
Crude death rate (CDR/1,000)	15.0	10.8	9.4	12.2
Infant mortality rate (IMR/1,000)	—	86 (1980)	66	80
Life expectancy at birth				
Males	49.1	55.7	58	53
Females	52.5	59.1	62	57
Total	50.8	57.4	61 (1990)	55
Annual growth rate	3.3 (1962–69)	3.0 (1969–82)	3.12 (1982–92)	2.53 (1978–97)
Rural vs. urban population (%)	—	R 74 U 26	R 69 U 31	R 68 U 32

— Not available.
Sources: As cited in Feresu, Nyandoro, and Mumbwanda 2000—adapted from CSO, June 1985, *National Health Strategy for Zimbabwe 1997–2005*, Harare; CSO, Nov. 1992, *Combined Demographic Analysis.*

slightly higher than the 69 percent recorded in 1994. Skilled delivery assistance for all live births also increased slightly in 1999, to 73 percent, from 69 percent in the 1994 ZDHS and 70 percent in the 1988 ZDHS. The skilled birth provider is primarily the midwife, who delivered 61, 57, and 59 percent of women in 1999, 1994, and 1988, respectively (CSO and MI 1989, 1995, 2000). Cesarean sections at 6.7 percent in 1999 are slightly higher than the 6.0 percent recorded in 1994, a proxy for met need. Antenatal care is nearly universal—with 93 percent of women receiving this care from a trained clinical professional for their most recent birth (80 percent with a trained nurse or midwife), according to the 1999 ZDHS. During the median 4.7 antenatal visits a woman receives, good quality care appears to be provided: 9 in 10 women had their blood pressure measured, 8 in 10 gave a urine sample and 3 in 4 a blood sample, 8 in 10 received a tetanus toxoid injection and 6 in 10 received iron tablets. Only 4 in 10 women, however, received information on the signs of pregnancy complications (CSO and MI 2000).

While urban women access the above services to a greater extent than their rural counterparts, 64 percent of rural women do use health facilities for birth and have a skilled birth attendant, and they have a cesarean section rate of 5.3 percent, according to the 1999 ZDHS. None of these rates vary greatly from those recorded in the 1994 ZDHS.

What Has Happened to Maternal Mortality in Zimbabwe?

The demographic and health surveys calculate the MMR based on a direct estimation using the sisterhood method. This looks at time of death (death during pregnancy or within two months postdelivery) without consideration of cause. However, the most likely explanation for the increase in the MMR is a change in the causes of maternal death.

Mbizvo reported causes in the 1989–90 community-based studies (Mbizvo and others 1994), based on medical diagnosis or maternal audit: 80 percent of maternal deaths were from such direct causes as hemorrhage, puerperal and postabortion sepsis, and hypertension or eclampsia; and only 20 percent were from indirect causes, including malaria and AIDS. While highly underreported and only reflecting hospital deaths, MOH data reveal an increasing proportion of maternal deaths from indirect causes, primarily malaria, AIDS-related problems, and cardiac failure. Better documented than maternal mortality are AIDS and AIDS-related deaths through MOH reporting as well as sentinel sites in both urban and rural areas. As figure 4.2 shows, there has been a steadily increasing trend in AIDS and AIDS-related conditions (ARC), including new cases of tuberculosis, beginning in 1993.

UNAIDS estimates that as of the end of 1999, 25 percent of adults (15–49 years) in Zimbabwe are living with HIV/AIDS

Figure 4.2 Zimbabwe: AIDS, ARC, and TB Cases, 1989–96

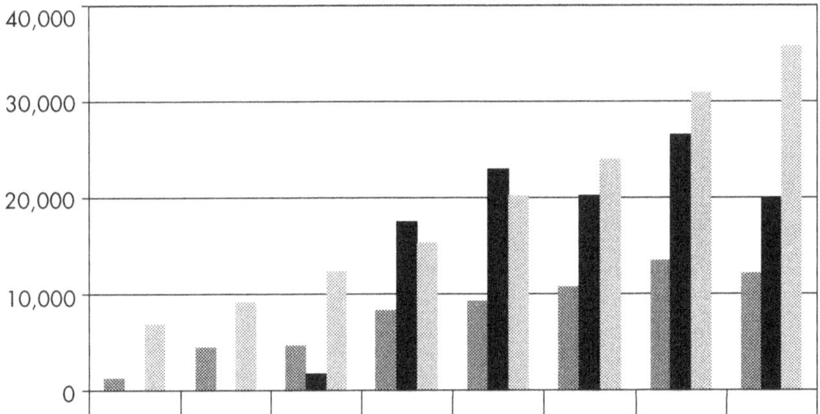

Cases	1989	1990	1991	1992	1993	1994	1995	1996
AIDS	1131	4362	4557	8180	9174	10647	13356	12029
ARC			1570	15237	22872	23959	26430	19780
TB	6812	9132	12198	17383	20125	20062	30831	35735

Note: AIDS = acquired immune deficiency syndrome, new cases; ARC = AIDS-related conditions, new cases; TB = tuberculosis, new cases.
Source: Zimbabwe Health Profile 1996, as cited in Feresu, Nyandoro, and Mumbwanda 2000.

(UNAIDS 2000). In the three major urban areas, HIV prevalence among tested antenatal clients increased from 10 percent in 1989 to 36 percent in 1994, then decreased to 30 percent in 1997. In 1997 a median of 30 percent of antenatal clients in 31 sentinel sites in rural areas tested positive for HIV. At these same sites, HIV prevalence among sexually transmitted disease (STD) clinic patients increased from 6 percent in 1987 to 72 percent in 1999 (UNAIDS 2000), as table 4.2 shows.

That AIDS is having an impact on maternal mortality ratios is becoming more obvious. Unofficial reports from Zambia and

Malawi also indicate a sharp increase in their respective MMRs over the past few years. In the University Teaching Hospital in Lusaka, Zambia, a two-year retrospective study of the etiology of all maternal deaths between January 1, 1996, and December 31, 1997, found that indirect causes contributed 58 percent of the maternal deaths, with most caused by malaria (30 percent) and tuberculosis and unspecified chronic respiratory tract infection, both linked primarily with AIDS (47 percent). As table 4.3 shows, the MMR in the hospital increased from 118 in 1982, to 667 in 1989, to 921 in 1996–97, primarily due to the increase in nonobstetric causes of death (Ahmed and others 1999).

Factors in Zimbabwe's Prior Success

Prior to this decade's reversal of the MMR, several factors contributed to Zimbabwe's reported low MMR:

- Policies aimed at equity, including a more equitable distribution of health services, were created.

- The infrastructure for health and family planning services was increased, decreasing geographic access issues.

- Financial access was ensured.

- Appropriate personnel were posted throughout the system.

- Efforts were made to link with the community through waiting mothers' shelters and traditional birth attendant programs.

Table 4.2 Zimbabwe: Prevalence of HIV by Group, 1999

GROUP	PERCENT
Adults (15–49 years)	25
Urban antenatal clients	30
31 sentinel sites—antenatal clients	30
31 sentinel sites—STD clients	72

Source: UNAIDS 2000.

Table 4.3 Zambia: Cause of Maternal Death, University Teaching Hospital, 1996–97

CAUSE	PERCENT
Direct	42
Indirect	58
Malaria	30
AIDS related	47
Tuberculosis	25
Unspecific chronic respiratory infection	22

Note: MMR 118 (1982); MMR 921 (1996–97).
Source: Ahmed and others 1999.

Creating Policy and Programs for Maternal Mortality Reduction

After independence in 1980, the Ministry of Health adopted the Primary Health Care (PHC) strategy as a way of closing the gap in the distribution of health services. The PHC strategy was realized through all levels from the provincial and district health services to the ward and village health committees in the community. One of the arms of PHC was maternal and child health, including family planning. The posting of the deputy secretary of health as its head denoted its importance.

Increasing Infrastructure

As a strategy to bring health to all and to correct the urban-rural imbalance, health facilities were constructed in large numbers, especially in the first postindependence decade. The number of health facilities increased by 37 percent overall from 1980 to 1997 (see table 4.4), with a 39 percent increase in the rural provinces compared with 20 percent in urban areas. Each of the 55 districts in the eight provinces of Zimbabwe has a district hospital and may have several rural hospitals and rural health centers as well. Each province has a provincial hospital, equipped to deal with most referrals from the respective district hospitals. At the tertiary level, there are six central hospitals, two in Harare and three in Bulawayo, the second largest city, and one in Chitungwiza, the third largest city. Three of these tertiary institutions, the two in Harare and one in Bulawayo, are also teaching hospitals. Today health services are offered through both the public and private sectors, including missions, rural councils, urban councils, private physicians, and mining and industrial health services. The ratio of population served by a hospital averages 48,000 to one in the provinces (minus the cities) and that by a clinic approximately 9,000 to one (table 4.5).

While this increase in health infrastructure was part of the response to the inequities noted preindependence, there was also a specific response to the 1987 launching of the Safe Motherhood Initiative: the government of Zimbabwe built eight district hospitals as a way of improving the infrastructure to respond to the maternal mortality problem noted.

Table 4.4 Zimbabwe: Number of Health Facilities, Pre-1980 and 1997

LOCATION	PRE-1980	1997	NUMBER (PERCENT)/INCREASE
Provinces			
Manicaland	104	238	134 (56.3)
Mashonaland Central	59	112	53 (47.3)
Mashonaland East	115	169	54 (32.0)
Mashonaland West	93	155	62 (40.0)
Matebeland North	68	89	21 (23.6)
Matebeland South	43	105	62 (59.0)
Midlands	167	213	46 (21.6)
Masvingo	115	165	50 (30.3)
Subtotal	764	1,246	482 (38.7)
Cities and towns			
Chitungwiza	2	4	2 (50.0)
Harare	39	54	15 (27.8)
Mutare	—	8	8 (100)
Gweru	—	—	—
Kwekwe	3	4	1 (25.0)
Bulawayo	27	19	−8 (−42.1)
Subtotal	71	89	18 (20.2)
Grand total	835	1,335	500 (37.5)

— Not available.
Source: Health Profiles 1997 as cited in Feresu, Nyandoro, and Mumbwanda 2000.

Table 4.5 Zimbabwe: Infrastructure by Population Level, 1997

LOCATION	POPULATION	HOSPITALS	POPULATION/ HOSPITAL	CLINICS	POPULATION/ CLINIC
Provinces					
Manicaland	1,814,764	40	45,369	219	8,287
Mashonaland Central	1,019,627	14	72,831	98	10,404
Mashonaland East	1,109,547	28	39,627	162	6,849
Mashonaland West	1,255,716	23	54,596	127	9,888
Masvingo	1,219,655	35	34,847	131	9,310
Matebeland North	683,917	17	40,230	75	9,119
Matebeland South	632,930	19	33,312	92	6,880
Midlands	1,510,150	32	47,193	191	7,907
Subtotal	9,952,595	208	47,849	1,095	9,089
Cities and towns					
Harare	1,219,655	7	174,236	41	29,748
Bulawayo	617,024	9	68,558	18	34,279
Grand total	11,789,274	224	52,630	1,154	10,216

Source: 1997 InterCensal Demographic Survey as cited in Feresu, Nyandoro, and Mumbwanda 2000.

Training and Posting Appropriate Personnel

The decade postindependence saw a major increase in health personnel. More nurses were trained in family planning and midwifery and deployed to the district and provincial hospitals. More nurses with a diploma in community nursing were trained to manage rural health services under the provincial and district medical officers of health. Trained personnel returned from overseas. This upward trend could not continue through the late 1990s; the numbers registered began to level off by mid-decade (figure 4.3). Even so, the numbers of midwives registered in 1997 would mean one available per population of 1,500. For nurses, the ratio would be one to 1,200. By the 1990s, the number of doctors could not fill all provincial posts; in 1997, only 80 percent were filled according to some MOH reports. Even so, MOH data show one doctor available for every 7,500 people.

Registration does not equal practicing, however, and with foreign or urban migration draining the ranks, the numbers of nurses, espe-

Figure 4.3 Zimbabwe: Midwives by Category, 1981–97

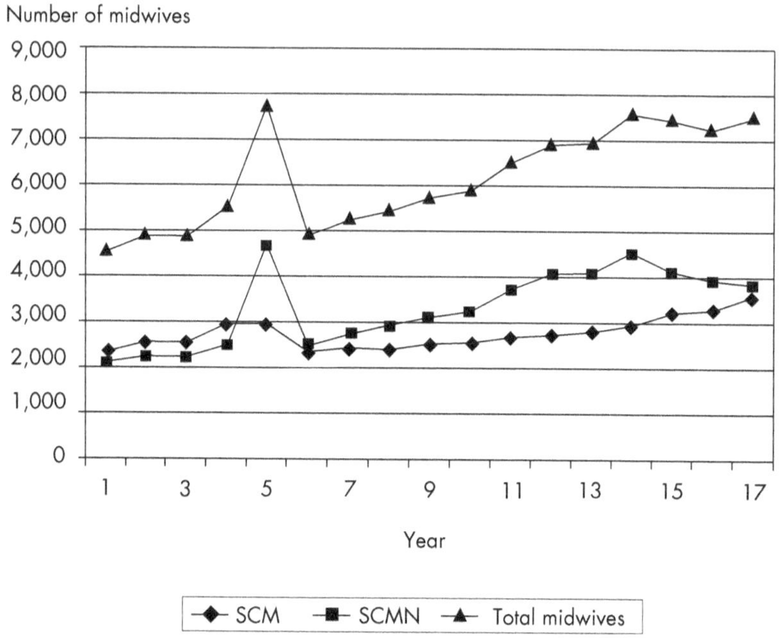

Number of midwives

[Line chart showing SCM, SCMN, and Total midwives from year 1 to year 17, with values ranging from about 2,000 to 8,000]

Note: SCM = state certified midwives; SCMN = state certified maternity nurses.
Sources: Health Professional Council of Zimbabwe; *Zimbabwe Epidemiological Bulletin*, no. 18; Ministry of Health reports 1988–1997, as cited in Feresu, Nyandoro, and Mumbwanda 2000.

cially nurse midwives in the periphery, are actually considered low. Table 4.6 on accessibility suggests that the level of staffing provided by the numbers registered is misleading. It is hoped that the new salary structure for the year 2000 will provide rural and responsibility allowances and so improve staffing in rural areas.

Registration does not necessarily equal skilled care either. To ensure skilled care during the first decade following independence, one strategy to reduce maternal mortality involved "appropriate" staffing at rural health centers. The establishment at a typical rural health center included two nurses (one a midwife), one nurse aide, and one groundskeeper or general hand.

Table 4.6 Zimbabwe: Nurses' Access Issues, 1999

LOCATION AND "BIG" PROBLEM	PERCENT
Urban	
Getting money for treatment	26.1
Fear of verbal abuse by provider	13.6
Rural	
Distance to a health facility	44.5
Have to take transport	43.0
Getting money for treatment	38.8
Not wanting to go alone	15.9
Fear of verbal abuse by provider	13.7

Source: CSO and MI 2000.

In 1986 the government started a program of attachment of nurses without midwifery for on-the-job training so they could deliver emergencies; it included a one-month attachment to a district maternity unit. The program is still ongoing because of attrition and the hiring of new employees. The total number of nurses who have undergone this program is not available. The MOH also enacted a policy in the first postindependence decade to promote nurses to high positions only if they had midwifery as well. Thus most nurse managers at district and provincial levels are also midwives.

Midwifery training includes one year in obstetrical care management for the most highly trained midwife, the state registered nurse (SRN); SRNs are equipped to practice on their own. They are trained to diagnose and manage complications during pregnancy and labor, perform a safe delivery, refer complicated cases, perform episiotomy, and deliver breech where necessary. SRNs can provide antibiotics, give sedatives, perform manual removal of placenta, resuscitate newborn infants, and give oxytocics—especially when these nurses function on their own in remote areas. During their training, they observe 10 deliveries and perform 20 deliveries. They are also taught to care for the newborn and for the mother and baby in the postnatal period.

The state certified midwife (SCM) and state certified maternity nurse (SCMN) are trained for only one year. For the latter, the course is geared to the first level of care, with more practice than theory provided. State certified nurses (SCN)—previously medical assistants—and SCMN mainly practice in rural health centers and clinic settings. Like the SCM, they can provide many of the bEOC functions (but not all), including give antibiotics, perform manual removal of placenta, resuscitate newborn infants, and give ergometrine postdelivery. Postindependence, SCN and SCMN who wished to upgrade their midwifery skills trained for another six months to a year. All nurses provide only institutional deliveries.

Implementing Maternity Services

Most hospitals and health centers throughout the country have delivery facilities, with maternity beds for antenatal admissions, deliveries, and postnatal services. While nurses and midwives are trained to carry out normal deliveries using a partograph, when they recognize problems, they refer to the next level. During antenatal screening, high-risk mothers may also be referred for delivery—that is, mothers with previous cesarean sections, high blood pressure, pregnancy-induced hypertension, multiple pregnancies, diabetes, or other medical conditions or previous intra- and postpartum complications, including hemorrhage, are referred to district, provincial, and central hospitals.

Cesarean sections are performed at central and provincial hospitals, but only some mission and district hospitals. The specific number of hospitals per province that can perform cesarean sections was not available.

Ensuring Access to Services

In 1988 the ZDHS reported that 85 percent of women of reproductive age lived within 8 kilometers of the nearest health facility and 100 percent had access to a hospital within 50–70 kilometers. While services for normal delivery are widely available, most women had to travel at least 30 kilometers for a cesarean section. Less than half of all women lived within 30 kilometers of a health facility with a maternity waiting home, a generator, or a blood bank. Quality of

Table 4.7 Zimbabwe: Impact of Family Planning Program, 1984–99

INDICATOR	1984	1988	1994	1999
Total fertility rate	6.5	5.5	4.3	4.0
Contraceptive prevalence rate (%)	38.4	43.1	48.0	54.0
Married women using methods (%)	27.0	36.0	42.0	53.5
Knowledge of modern methods (%)				
Women 15–49 years	82.8	96.3	99.0	96.8
Men 18–55 years	—	98.3	99.0	99.1

— Not available.
Sources: *Strategy for the Zimbabwe Family Planning Council* for the five years from 1997 to 2002, as cited in Feresu, Nyandoro, and Mumbwanda 2000; CSO and MI 2000.

care needed improvement, as health services were considered too far, with long waiting times, discourteous service, and drug shortages (CSO and MI 1989).

By 1999 the ZDHS reports that the majority of women in both rural and urban areas did not perceive a problem with knowing where to go, getting permission, or doing without a female service provider. As table 4.6 shows, 25 percent of urban women did see getting the money for treatment as a problem, as did 39 percent of rural women. Rural women also considered transport and lack of a nearby facility to be major problems (43 and 45 percent, respectively). Fourteen percent of all women feared verbal abuse by the health service provider (CSO and MI 2000).

Increasing the Availability of Family Planning Services in Rural Areas

Although mortality appears to be on the rise, fertility continues to decline in Zimbabwe. Today on average a woman will have 4 children, as opposed to 5.5 children in 1988 (table 4.7). As of the 1999 ZDHS, 54 percent of women were using a method of contraception, showing a steady trend upward from the 48 and 43 percent use of contraceptives in 1994 and 1988, respectively (CSO and MI 1989, 1995, 2000). In 1999 knowledge of modern methods was increasing faster than overall use, with the greatest increase in knowledge of injectable contraceptives. Knowledge of family planning has been universal since 1994 across all subgroups.

When family planning programs began in 1953, services were confined to the mainly white community in the urban areas. In 1965, the Family Planning Association of Rhodesia was formed, coordinating the scattered family planning services; in 1966 the MOH approved these services for provision through government hospitals and clinics, opening services for the total population (though in a very limited way). By the mid-1970s, 28 family planning clinics existed. In 1976 the association initiated a community-based program for distribution of pills and condoms. The Zimbabwe National Family Planning Council (ZNFPC) was formed as a parastatal in 1984 under the MOH. By 1987 its outreach program, which included the use of mobile clinics, covered 29 percent of the rural population (CSO and MI 1989). Today mobile clinics are far less utilized.

Now family planning constitutes an integral part of maternal and child health in Zimbabwe, with most health facilities offering some methods. Government services provide 65 percent of all methods, ZNFPC 9 percent, and missions, private sector services, and others the rest. Community-based distributors (CBD) provide only 7 percent of the total. All methods are available (including Norplant, the female condom, and emergency contraception); the pill and condom are available through the CBD program in the rural areas.

Abortion is permitted if continuation of the pregnancy threatens the woman's life or permanent impairment of her physical health, or if there is serious risk that the child would suffer from grave physical or mental defects. It is also permitted in cases of rape or incest or if the woman is mentally handicapped. However, physician or legal consent must be secured first.

While reliable national estimates of induced abortion are not readily available, government reports suggest that abortions may have been on the rise since 1996.

Establishing Waiting Mothers' Shelters

Maternity waiting mothers' shelters (WMS) are residential facilities located near a qualified medical facility, where women defined as high risk can await their deliveries. The waiting mothers' shelters

Table 4.8 Zimbabwe: Waiting Mothers' Shelters by Province, 1996–97

PROVINCE	NUMBER OF WMS	EXPECTED PREGNANT WOMEN/ YEAR	EXPECTED PREGNANT WOMEN/ WMS	MATERNAL MORTALITY RATIO IN 1997	POPULATION OF WOMEN/ PER PROVINCE 1997
Manicaland	59	84,332	1,429	153.8	954,566
Mashonaland Central	13	47,800	3,677	200.7	524,088
Mashonaland East	15	56,994	3,800	62.2	596,936
Mashonaland West	27	54,520	2,019	133.6	647,949
Masvingo	59	53,529	907	110.1	656,174
Matebeland North	26	35,600	1,369	75.4	356,321
Matebeland South	29	30,693	1,058	126	339,883
Midlands	27	64,183	2,377	139.1	797,359
Total	255	427,651	16,636	n.a.	4,873,276

n.a. Not applicable.
Note: WMS = waiting mothers' shelters. Population excludes Harare (1,871,943) and Bulawayo (671,024). WMS is calculated as expected pregnant women divided by number of waiting mother's shelters.
Source: Ministry of Health Reports 1997, as cited in Feresu, Nyandoro, and Mumbwanda 2000.

were originally established before independence by mission hospitals, which realized that in the third trimester, a rural woman needs to be near a delivery facility.

The WMS are supposed to be built where there is a means of communication (radio links or telephones) for accessing the referral unit. Most districts and provinces began to construct or upgrade waiting mothers' shelters after 1994. Table 4.8 shows the distribution of the shelters by province in 1996–97.

Analysis of responses to a questionnaire from four of the provinces clearly reveals that the MOH's plan for the WMS has not been fully implemented. A good proportion of the health facilities do not include a midwife to supervise the shelter, nor do they all have means of communications with which to check for advice or send for referral.

Calling Perinatal Mortality Meetings

Perinatal mortality meetings are a periodic feature in the Greater Harare Unit, which comprises the Harare maternity hospital and the city of Harare clinics. During the first decade postindependence these meetings were expanded to staff managers in provincial and district services. These meetings aim to ensure quality and are educational as well as supervisory. The coverage of home-based maternal deaths is low, however. It is hoped that with the introduction of a new maternal mortality form requesting details of the death and care, and more-focused perinatal mortality meetings, more home-based deaths will be captured.

Establishing a Traditional Midwives Program

According to the 1999 ZDHS, traditional birth attendants deliver nearly 18 percent of births, similar to the levels reported in the 1994 ZDHS (17 percent), but up substantially from the 6 percent in the 1988 ZDHS. Zimbabwe started a traditional midwives (TM) program that continues to date under the provincial health services. The district-nursing officer supervises TMs and the rural health center nurse upgrades their skills. Supervisory meetings are planned for each month at the local health centers.

Before 1987, TM training fell to the community worker and was not standardized. TMs' training is now standardized using an MOH-WHO manual. TMs practice deliveries during their six-week training with instructors who are either SCM or SCMN. This training is practical and aims to upgrade the TMs' skills by building on what they already know. Part of the course covers recognition of complications during pregnancy and labor and where to refer (a local health center). On average, each traditional midwife delivers about two babies a year. They are instructed to bring mother and baby to the clinic for postdelivery checkups and registration.

Economic Impact on the Health Care System

The amount of money spent by public authority for each person in Zimbabwe has oscillated over the past two decades: it increased consistently in the 1980s up to Z$59 per capita in 1990–91, then dropped to Z$36 in 1995–96 and increased to Z$41 in 1996–97. The increase in the amount spent per person, however, does not take into account the depreciation of the Zimbabwe dollar and high inflation. There has been a real decrease in the health expenditure in the 1990s.

In 1991, in an effort to reform Zimbabwe's economy, the country initiated the World Bank's Economic Structural Adjustment Program (ESAP). Services now carry charges to the patient. Postindependence, a policy of hospital and clinic fee exemptions for those earning Z$150 a month or less has been instituted. Most people in rural areas obtained free medical services. In the early 1990s the amount was increased to Z$400 a month. However, user fees as a means of cost recovery were introduced in urban areas in the mid-1990s and in rural areas in 1998, as a result of the ESAP.

After conducting interviews with health center providers in one of the districts, Feresu and her colleagues stated, "The introduction of antenatal care and delivery fees was a sore point for the community, especially when there were no drugs" (2000, p. 71). While there has been an effort to ensure essential drugs in Zimbabwe, a critical shortage is now being experienced. The problem, according to Feresu and her colleagues, is with the delay in payment of tenders by government, which has resulted in refusals by private companies to supply drugs without cash upfront.

Conclusion

In the first decade postindependence, many interventions directed at improving health care of the Zimbabwean population were implemented, with a positive effect on maternal mortality. However, a reduction in the government health allocation in real terms, the increasing gap between the rich and poor social strata, and the ravaging HIV/AIDS epidemic have combined to worsen the health status of Zimbabweans since, with tragic effect on the MMR.

References

Ahmed, Yusef, P. Mwaba, C. Chintu, J. M. Grange, A. Ustianowski, and A. Zumla. 1999. "A Study of Maternal Mortality at the University Teaching Hospital, Lusaka, Zambia: The Emergence of Tuberculosis as a Major Non-Obstetric Cause of Maternal Death." *International Journal of Tuberculosis and Lung Disease* 3(8):675–80.

CSO (Central Statistical Office) (Zimbabwe) and MI (Macro International Inc.). 1989. *Zimbabwe Demographic and Health Survey, 1988*. Calverton, Md.: CSO and MI.

———. 1995. *Zimbabwe Demographic and Health Survey, 1994*. Calverton, Md.: CSO and MI.

———. 2000. *Zimbabwe Demographic and Health Survey, 1999*. Calverton, Md.: CSO and MI.

Feresu, A. S., with M. Nyandoro and L. Mumbwanda. 2000. *A Case Study of Maternal Mortality Trends in Zimbabwe, 1980–1997*. Prepared for the John Snow, Inc. Research and Training Institute.

Mbizvo, M. T., S. Fawcus, G. Lindmark, L. Nystrom, and the Maternal Mortality Study Group. 1994. *A Community-Based Study of Maternal Mortality in Zimbabwe*. Harare: University of Zimbabwe.

UNAIDS. 2000. "Zimbabwe UNAIDS/WHO Epidemiological Fact Sheet." www.unaids.org.

PART 2

Research Studies

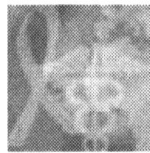
CHAPTER 5

Bolivia, 1996–2000

*Guillermo Seoane, Ramiro Equiluz,
Miguel Ugalde, and Juan Carlos Arraya*

Health care costs in Bolivia were assumed to be a major impediment to the use of services, such as a skilled birth attendant and a hospital for birthing. To overcome this barrier and reduce the MMR of 390 per 100,000 live births (INE and MI 1994), a national health insurance plan has been phased in to cover the costs of services vital to the reduction of maternal and infant mortality. In July 1996 the Bolivian government implemented the National Maternal and Child Health Insurance (MCHI) Program, with the main objective, as the name implies, of increasing coverage of maternal and child care. For pregnant women and babies, the insurance covered prenatal, labor and delivery, and postpartum and newborn care, including cesarean sections and coverage for other obstetrical emergencies. On December 31, 1998, the government created the Basic Health Insurance (BHI) to augment the MCHI, with explicit coverage of complications of pregnancy, delivery, and postpartum, including postabortion care, along with coverage for complications of the newborn, sexually transmitted infections, malaria, tuberculosis, and cholera. Whereas the MCHI covers 26 services, the BHI covers 76. The BHI also covers some laboratory tests, transfer of referred patients in cases of obstetric emergencies, regular visits by health personnel to rural communities without health facilities, and the printing of forms. It extends coverage beyond the public sector to Social Security, selected NGOs, and church-dependent facilities. Funding rates were increased to cover services and provide an incentive for priority interventions (for example, for delivery, a third of the reimbursement rate corresponds to an added incentive), and administrative procedures were streamlined.

The WHO Mother-Baby Package guides the protocols used for management of the problems covered by the maternity services under the BHI. Facilities are reimbursed on a per-service rate set annually by the MOH. These funds, dispersed by the municipalities, cover drugs, supplies, hospitalization, and laboratory exams associated with the covered services. Labor and equipment are covered by the central government and municipalities, respectively, and are not part of the insurance. The BHI is financed by a fixed 6.4 percent of municipality funds received from the central government's tax revenue, as initially stipulated by the Law of Popular Participation (1994). These funds are provided on a per capita basis and deposited into a special BHI account at the municipality level, the Local Compensatory Health Fund. Funds that accumulate cannot be used for other services but can carry over to the following year.

Increase in Use of Skilled Birth Attendants

According to the demographic and health surveys, the use of skilled birth assistance (such as doctors and nurses) increased nationally from the time before the MCHI went into effect (1994) to just after (1998)—from 47 percent in 1994 (INE and MI 1994) to 59 percent in 1998 (INE and MI 1998), an increase of nearly a quarter over the four years (the percentages relate to births in the previous three years) (table 5.1). In rural areas between 1994 and 1998, the use of skilled delivery rose by more than a quarter, from 26 to 34 percent, while urban percentages saw an increase of a little less than a fifth, from 66 to 78 percent. More deliveries were reported as taking place in facilities (42 percent in 1994 rising to 56 percent in 1999), but obviously some deliveries with skilled care are still being done in the home. Cesarean section rates have increased by nearly two-fifths to 15 percent from 11 percent (1998 versus 1994), with the rise primarily among women in the urban areas—21 percent from 15 percent

Table 5.1 Bolivia: Use of Maternity Care, 1989–2000

INDICATOR	YEAR (PERCENT)						
	1989	1994	1996	1997	1998	1999	2000
Facility delivery: DHS	—	42.2	—	—	55.9	—	—
Facility delivery: SNIS	—	—	16.9	22.1	22.5	22.5	27.4
Delivery with skilled birth attendant: DHS	43.2	47.1	—	—	59.3	—	—
Delivery with skilled birth attendant: SNIS	—	—	22.3	25.8	26.5	30	31.6
Cesarean section: DHS	—	10.6	—	—	14.7	—	—
Cesarean section: SNIS	—	—	2.8	3.6	4.1	4.9	5.5

— Not available.
Note: Use of SNIS data by year proportionately increased to 100 percent of reports. Percent of all facilities reporting: 1996—80.62 percent; 1997—81.49 percent; 1998—89.71 percent; 1999—90.55 percent; 2000—86.99 percent.
Source: Seoane and others 2000.

urban versus 6.0 from 5.9 percent in rural areas (table 5.1) (INE and MI 1994, 1998).

An examination of these same data by quintile of socioeconomic status (based on assets or wealth) (Gwatkin and others 2000) reveals that the poorest quintile showed the greatest improvement in using skilled care for birthing—rising nearly twofold from 11 percent in 1994 to 20 percent in 1998. Obviously this quintile also had, and continues to have, the greatest room for improvement. The fourth and fifth quintiles, the richest, had the least to achieve, as 75 percent and 99 percent, respectively, were already using skilled delivery care in 1994 (rising to 88 percent and 98 percent in 1998). Overall, most of the increase was in the use of doctors versus nurse-midwives for delivery (53 percent were assisted by doctors in 1998 versus 43 percent in 1994; nurse-midwives covered 5 percent of births in 1994 and only 4 percent in 1998). Among the poorest quintile use of public facilities increased the most (from 7 to 14 percent), while among the richest use of private facilities increased (although about half of this group still uses public facilities).

Government reporting (SNIS) is markedly lower than DHS information concerning use of facilities (any kind) for births, cesarean section rate (population-based), and use of skilled birth attendants (table 5.1). The SNIS information clearly reveals that many health providers give skilled birth care in the home; from the DHS data, this difference between facility and provider coverage is not as wide. According to Dmytraczenko, the percentage of maternal services being delivered by secondary and tertiary facilities has increased, while the opposite is true at the primary level. Patients are increasingly seeking care at higher-level facilities, where they perceive better quality of care. Unfortunately, services in these facilities are also more expensive because of the higher labor costs of specialists, who also tend to prescribe more advanced diagnostics and treatments, as well as other costs of labor, utilities, and building maintenance (Dmytraczenko and others n.d.).

The Impact of Insurance on Use of Services

In an evaluation of the MCHI, a study found that there was substantial growth in use of prenatal care and inpatient births, services covered by insurance, compared with use of other services not covered by insurance (see table 5.2) (Dmytraczenko and others n.d.). Prenatal visits increased in public facilities by 39 percent compared with 29 percent for other outpatients, and total births by 50 percent versus 26 percent for other types of inpatients. At the same time, the

Table 5.2 Bolivia: Growth in Utilization after the National Maternal and Child Health Insurance (MCHI) Program

	FACILITY (PERCENT)			
SERVICE	PUBLIC	SOCIAL SECURITY	NGO	PRIVATE
Total prenatal visits	39	16	94	−50
Other outpatients	29	34	61	−56
Total births	50	43	28	−37
Other inpatients	26	18	47	−29

Note: The percent change was determined by records: 18 months post-MCHI minus 18-month period pre-MCHI. MCHI was implemented July 1996.
Source: Dmytraczenko and others n.d.

private sector saw a decrease in patients. Numbers of patients refer to those reported in the SNIS for the 18-month period pre-MCHI and the 18-month period post-MCHI.

The analysis by quintile shows that the poorest segment of the population has increased use of skilled birth attendants and of health facilities for birthing. However, the poorest segment has the longest way to go to be covered by a skilled provider in birth: as of 1998, approximately 80 percent of the poorest were still outside of services. Most of the insurance funds are covering the costs of those better off, nearly all of them using skilled care for birthing.

Pros and Cons of the Insurance

While increases in service use have been reported, there is obviously room for improvement. Through interviews and focus groups with both users and providers, possible gaps in implementation of insurance schemes have been determined.

The Clients' Perspective

Information about the new insurance, BHI, is not universal. In 2000, in exit interviews with 180 women using either prenatal or postpartum care at one of the three levels of care (referral hospital, district hospital, health center) in one of three areas (La Paz, Cochabamba, Santa Cruz), 42 percent said they had not had any information on the insurance scheme. Among those who had received information, nearly half stated they had gotten it from the health provider, while another 40 percent learned about the BHI from television or radio. About half of those interviewed knew that BHI covered prenatal and delivery services, but only 12 percent knew it covered postpartum care.

User satisfaction with the insured services was high; 65 percent stated that the quality of care had improved. For a quarter of these women, this improvement was related to services having no or low fees; another 9 percent found services improved because they could now get free medicines. More than 90 percent of all those interviewed felt they were treated well and received a careful medical examination. A quarter of the women mentioned, however, that the health personnel did not explain anything. Nearly half of the interviewed women felt they had to wait too long, which seemed to be related to waiting more than one hour. Approximately a third of women stated that they had suffered some type of complication. Over 90 percent of these said they had had it resolved favorably; more than 50 percent were treated for their complication within 30 minutes of arrival. Some 85 percent of interviewed women said they were satisfied with the attention they received, and 95 percent stated they would return because they had received good care (43 percent) or needed a follow-up visit (40 percent); only 9 percent said they would return because services are free. Clients used the services because of the close location, familiarity, and relatives' recommendations (Dmytraczenko and others 1998) and the advice from the health worker counseling (Seoane and others 2000).

While public facility registration and services are supposedly free, 12 percent of women interviewed paid for registration, and 46 percent stated they had paid for services (primarily ultrasound and lab analysis) and medicines; most paid between $b10 and $b99. Medications may still require personal payment because the drugs may not be available at the health facility. The list of medications covered by the BHI encompasses 83 products for the three levels of care (excluding the surgery room list). Approximately half of the women interviewed had also gone to private services, where 40 percent of them spent up to $b10 but another 40 percent spent up to $b999.

The Providers' Perspective

Among the 72 doctors, nurses, and nurse auxiliaries interviewed in 2000 from all levels of care in the three municipalities of La Paz, Cochabamba, and Santa Cruz, 75 percent agreed with the establishment of the BHI, although most wanted minor changes. Slightly more than half felt that the insurance improved the quality of care, with the majority stating that they agreed with the established treatments in the BHI protocols. Theoretical training on the protocols was received by only half, however, primarily nurses and nurse-auxiliaries at the first and second levels of care. Only a quarter of all interviewed had received practical training, most of these at the primary level of care. Providers at the tertiary facilities received little to no training on the BHI protocols.

Three-quarters of the providers interviewed had experienced stockouts for some BHI listed drugs (this was most apparent in Santa Cruz and at second and tertiary levels of care). This perhaps underestimates the problem as no facility was found to have all supplies on the list. Upon observation at three different health posts, the average deficit of the 57 essential drugs on the BHI list for that level of care was 46 percent. At health-center level, the observations found wide variation in the drug list deficit; for example, one was missing only 15 percent of the 83 BHI drugs for the HC level, while another was missing 85 percent. District hospitals had between 15 and 27 percent of the 94 BHI drugs for their level missing. Even the three referral hospitals observed had between 13 and 63 percent of their 94 listed drugs missing. In cases of stockout, the most frequent response is to ask the patient to pay at a private pharmacy. The reason for stockouts was primarily lack of insurance reimbursement, which was also noted in the MCHI evaluation of 1998.

The BHI requires new administrative procedures, yet less than a third of those providers interviewed had received any training in the procedures and only about 60 percent had access to the procedures manual. Three-quarters stated they had the necessary registration forms; opinion was split as to whether the forms required much time to fill out.

Problems with the BHI were primarily lack of information about the users of BHI, timely availability of drugs, lack of human resources, and delays in payment.

Conclusions

The national health insurance plans, the MCHI and the BHI, have been associated with an increase in the use of skilled care, although the level of use among the poorest quintile remains troubling at less than 20 percent in 1998. Obvious steps for improvement include providing readily accessible information to families (especially those most difficult to reach—the indigenous and remote), improving the drug supply, and ensuring timely payment for services rendered. Not so easily remedied would be improving the quality of care provided, which is already perceived by clients and providers as having improved (though competency-based training was not the norm for hospital personnel), reaching the unreached, and addressing the public-private mix. Bolivia's indigenous population constitutes more than half the total population; diversity in languages as well as traditions of health and health care makes this population particularly challenging to reach.

Why did the insurance work to improve coverage with a skilled birth attendant? The answer is, probably by addressing a felt need by a portion of the population to access services. It probably did not act through changing behaviors among families or among providers as efforts to reach out were minimal in the first phase of the insurance plan.

References

Dmytraczenko, Tania, I. Aitken, S. C. Carrasco, K. C. Seoane, J. Holley, W. B. Abramson, A. S. Valle, and M. A. Effen. 1998. *Evaluacion del Seguro Nacional de Maternidad y Ninez en Bolivia. Informe technico No. 22*. Bethesda, Md.: Abt Associates Inc.

Dmytraczenko, Tania, S. Scribner, C. Leighton, and K. Novak. No date. "Delivering Priority Health Services to Poor Mothers and Children." *PHR Executive Summary Series* 1–8.

Gwatkin, D. R., S. Rutstein, K. Johnson, R. Pande, and A. Wagstaff. 2000. *Socio-Economic Differences in Health, Nutrition, and Population in Bolivia*. The World Bank. HNP Publication Series, HNP/Poverty Thematic Group. World Bank, Washington, D.C.

INE (Instituto Nacional de Estadistica) (Bolivia) and MI (Macro International Inc.). 1994. *Bolivia Encuesta Nacional de Demografia y Salud, 1994*. Calverton, Md.: CBS and MI.

———. 1998. *Bolivia Encuesta Nacional de Demografia y Salud, 1998*. Calverton, Md.: CBS and MI.

Seoane, Guillermo, Ramiro Eguiluz, Miguel Ugalde, and Juan Carlos Arraya. 2000. *Improvement on Women's Health Care Due to the Health Reform in Bolivia*. Report prepared for the John Snow, Inc. Research and Training Institute.

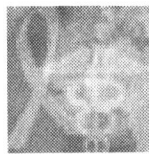

CHAPTER 6

Egypt, 1992–2000
Oona Campbell

Egypt shows evidence of maternal mortality decline over the past 25 years (table 6.1). The most comprehensive studies are the national maternal mortality study (NMMS) in 1992–93 and the more recent NMMS in 2000, which show there has been a dramatic decline in maternal mortality between 1992–93 and 2000 from 174 per 100,000 live births to below 84 per 100,000 (MOH 1994; MOHP 2001). Currently, metropolitan Egypt has the lowest proportion of maternal deaths (5.1 percent), followed by Lower Egypt, Upper Egypt, and frontier (7.8 percent, 8.9 percent, and 15.8 percent, respectively). Although all methods are likely to miss some maternal deaths, the use of the same approach in both studies means the degree of underestimation is likely to be similar.

Where Women Deliver and Who Delivers Them

Egypt has for some time had a large number of medical doctors and a considerable health infrastructure (Sayed 1991). Figure 6.1 shows that the percent of births attended by a skilled attendant (doctor or nurse) has increased from 11 percent in 1977 to 40 percent in 1990 to 61 percent in 1998. These skilled attendants are largely obstetricians (82 percent of skilled attendants), who may hold one of several degrees: the diploma, which consists primarily of a one-year theoretical course; the M.S., which consists of a minimum of two years, the first part on basic sciences and theses or essays on obstetrics-gynecology-related problems; the M.D., which consists of a mini-

Table 6.1 Egypt: Population-Based Studies of Maternal Mortality, 1963–2000

LOCATION	YEAR	NUMBER OF MATERNAL DEATHS	MMR	REFERENCE
Lower Egypt				
Giza study	1985–86	153	150	El Kady and others 1989
Menoufia (RAMOS)	1981–83	385	190	Fortney and others 1984, 1986
Alexandria	1963–82	183	163	El Ghamry and others 1984
Upper Egypt				
Assiut (Kausaih)	1984–85	16	178	Abdullah and others 1985
Sohag	1984–85	23	471	Abdullah and others 1985
Qena	1984–85	34	323	Abdullah and others 1985
Assiut + 3 villages	1987–88	29	368	Abdullah and others 1992
National				
National Sisterhood method estimate[a]	≈ 1976	150	170	Stanton, Abderrahim, and Hill 1997
National Sisterhood method estimate[a]	≈ 1979	87	177	Abdel-Azeem, Farid, and Khalifa 1993
Urban	≈ 1979	n.s.	150	Abdel-Azeem, Farid, and Khalifa 1993
Rural	≈ 1979	n.s.	193	Abdel-Azeem, Farid, and Khalifa 1993
National Maternal Mortality Study[a]	1992–93	772	174	MOH 1994
Rapid Assessment Survey	1997	n.s.	96	MOHP 1997
National Maternal Mortality Study	2000	585	<100	MOHP 2001

n.s. Not stated.
a. Excluding frontier governorates.

mum of two more years of academic research after the M.S.; the MRCOG, which consists of three years of practical training; and the Egyptian Board degree for obstetrics-gynecology, which is a practical, on-the-job degree for Ministry of Health and Population (MOHP) employees (Adel Hakim Issa and Hussein Samy, personal communications, 2001; Fahmy 1988). Midwives compose 17 percent of skilled attendants while general practitioners (GPs) are 3 percent. Births by TBAs (dayas) and relatives have decreased accord-

Figure 6.1 Egypt: Percentage of Births by Facility and Attendant, 1976–98

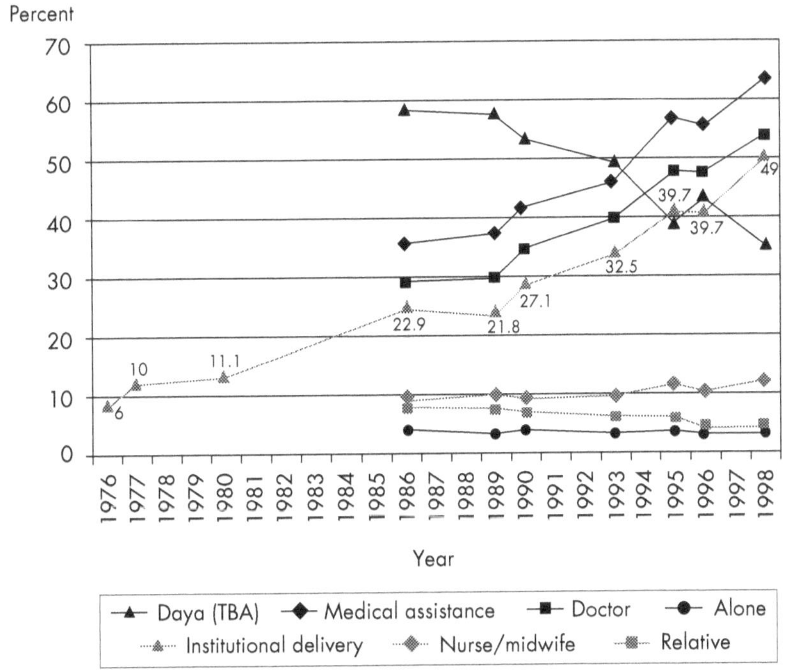

Legend: Daya (TBA); Medical assistance; Doctor; Alone; Institutional delivery; Nurse/midwife; Relative

Source: CAPMAS 1987; WHO 1993; El Zanaty and Way 2001.

ingly. Figure 6.1 also shows that the proportion of births occurring in health facilities has increased from 6 percent in 1976 to 27 percent in 1990 to 49 percent in 1998.

In the period from the 1992–93 NMMS to the 2000 NMMS, Egypt appears to have moved away from being a Model 1, in which home births and TBA deliveries predominate. Currently, none of the other models (2–4) have a majority of births. Doctors, and to a lesser extent midwives, attend births at home, in private clinics, in MCH centers, in bEOC facilities, and in public and private cEOC facilities. Much of the expansion in facility births has been in the private sector, which has increased from about a third of facility births to slightly over half. In the five years prior to 2000, health facility births in the private sector have overtaken births in the public sector, 26 to 22 percent, respectively (El-Zanaty and Way 2001).

Policy Guiding Action

This change appears to be in part the result of late 1960s and early 1970s policies to expand medical education and increase the numbers of doctors, though these policies do not seem to relate specifically to maternity care. There were also deliberate policies to close midwifery schools in the early 1970s. However, in 1995, the MOH issued a decree licensing midwifery training once again, and pilot programs were started on a small scale. In addition, the following year, health sector reform efforts to rationalize (reduce) the number of physicians and increase the number of nurses got underway (Sallam 1998). There appear to be no MOH policies about where births should take place, or whether the MOH wants to encourage private sector deliveries.

The policy approach to dayas (traditional birth attendants) has also varied. In 1912 Egypt's first daya school was opened; by the 1930s, health centers had daya schools attached. However, in 1954 the government issued a decree to gradually abolish these schools, and by 1962 all had been closed (Hefni and Kassas 1991). Etman and colleagues (1984) note that in 1969, the Egyptian Ministry of Health, confident that sufficient numbers of trained nurses and nurse-midwives were available, revoked the licensure of indigenous dayas. Despite these legal restrictions, dayas at that time attended over 90 percent of deliveries in Egypt. Since the early 1980s, however, activities aimed at training dayas, rather than excluding them, have been undertaken, including programs under the auspices of UNICEF and the Child Spacing Program of the Egypt Ministry of Health (Ricter 1992; UNICEF 1985). These have emphasized avoiding harmful practices and the early detection and referral of women with obstetric complications. Despite such training, dayas clearly have a diminishing role today; in 2000, they did only 36 percent of deliveries (El-Zanaty and Way 2001). Furthermore, studies show that although most dayas learned their skills from their mothers, few expect their daughters to learn their trade from them.

Dayas are primarily expected to refer complications; they were found to contribute substandard care in only 8 percent of maternal deaths. These results may also indicate that the Ministry of Health and Population and UNICEF were relatively successful in training traditional birth attendants to promptly refer women who have complications.

Access to Emergency Care

Egypt has a well-developed infrastructure of facilities and roads that facilitate access to obstetric care in case of emergency. The country's high population density also means that most women live within close reach of medical facilities. Data from a 1989 survey on availability of services suggest that even in rural areas, 99 percent of women live within 30 kilometers of at least one government hospital (Sayed 1991). Since then there have been improvements in roads and hospital functioning. Most women with complications appear to be able to access emergency care. The 2000 NMMS shows that 93 percent of women accessed medical care at some point during the events leading to their deaths.

Review of maternal deaths reveals evidence that there was no proper referral system in place and that the problem concerns both where and when to refer cases. The first medical provider's failure to refer correctly was associated with 13 percent of deaths. In a disproportionately large number of cases, private practitioners delayed referring women to hospital facilities. In addition, even though most women (93 percent) saw a medical provider, only 62 percent of maternal deaths occurred in health facilities; 29 percent occurred at home, and 9 percent occurred during transportation. A slightly worrisome feature is that around a quarter of women delivering in facilities died at home or during transportation (27 percent for those delivering in private facilities and 23 percent for those delivering in public facilities). This suggests possible problems with referrals or

Figure 6.2 Egypt: Percentage of Births with Cesarean Section, 1976–2000

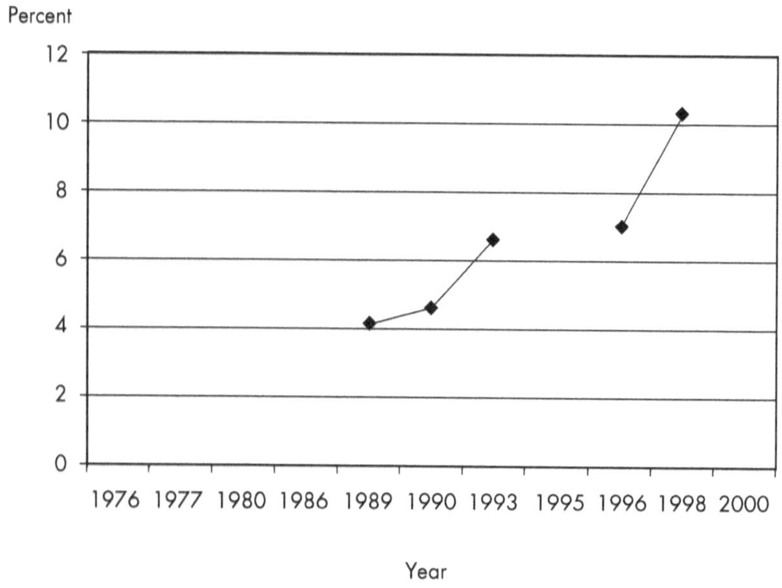

Source: Abdel-Azeem, Farid, and Khalifa 1993; El-Zanaty and Way 2000.

premature discharge. Furthermore, midwives do around 7 percent of deliveries and GPs normally do around 1 percent of deliveries but were found to contribute to 4 percent and 11 percent of maternal deaths, respectively. The relatively large contribution of GPs to deaths suggests either that they are engaged in harmful practices or that they are not properly stabilizing or referring emergency cases. This is an area that needs more research and policy decisionmaking.

With the exception of blood, the lack of appropriate facilities does not prevent many women from getting care. The lack of blood banks was the leading contributor (16 percent) to maternal death, followed by distance (4 percent), lack of transportation (5 percent), or the two together (7 percent). Lack of drugs (2 percent), supplies (2 percent), and equipment (5 percent) in health facilities contributed to 6 percent of maternal deaths. Lack of available operating rooms, backup facilities, and anesthetists and anesthetic facilities contributed to 2 percent, 2 percent, and 4 percent of maternal deaths, respectively. However, the small contribution of such factors was already the case in 1992. Nonetheless, the Ministry of Health and Population has been upgrading delivery facilities, and in the late 1990s, basic and comprehensive essential obstetric care services standards, essential obstetric care physical facility structural specifications, an essential obstetric care commodity catalog, and comprehensive essential surgical care physical facility structural specifications were defined (MOHP 2000, n.d.).

Cesarean section rates are within the 5 to 15 percent recommended by UNICEF and WHO as an indicator of met need for cesarean sections (figure 6.2). However, these figures need to be interpreted cautiously as they may also be an indicator of overmedicalized services.

Little data were available on cost as a financial barrier to emergency care. In 1996 a new cost recovery program was introduced in all hospitals, but health care services are meant to be provided freely throughout the country when needed (Sallam 1998).

Quality of Care

Since the 1992–93 NMMS (MOH 1994) report drew attention to the substandard care provided by obstetricians, several efforts have been underway to improve the quality of delivery care. The National Child Survival Project (1990–96), MotherCare Egypt Project (1996–98), UNICEF project (1996–present), and Healthy Mother/Healthy Child Project (1998–present) have targeted maternal and neonatal mortality through interventions to improve the use and quality of antenatal, delivery, and postpartum health services. The first project was national; the other three projects focused on Upper Egypt where mortality levels were highest.

If judged by the reduction in maternal mortality, quality of care has obviously improved, probably via increased access and use of skilled attendant and emergency care. However, in 2000 poor care by obstetricians still played a major role in the avoidable factors contributing to maternal death, with failure of early diagnosis and poor management contributing to 19 percent and 42 percent of all deaths, respectively.

In 1992, the fact emerged that sometimes no protocols for dealing with obstetric emergencies existed; most of these emergencies were managed by junior staff, with senior staff usually called too late (El Mouelhy 1987). Although the MOHP has now introduced protocols and standards for managing 10 common obstetric emergencies (such as postpartum hemorrhage) in Upper Egypt (MOHP 2000, n.d.), these are not as yet widespread throughout the country. Obstetric and core care protocols have also been developed for normal pregnancy and delivery and antenatal and postnatal care (MotherCare Egypt 1998; MOHP 2000). Competency-based training modules based on clinical protocols and standards have also been developed and tested. Training programs have been designed and tested for master and physician trainers (MotherCare Egypt 1998; MOHP n.d.).

Another problem to emerge is the increasing proportion of deaths in which medically trained providers have administered harmful treatments. These appear most marked with the use of oxytocic drugs and increased proportions of ruptured uteruses seen. In addition, national cesarean section rates are increasing, suggesting the potential for iatrogenic deaths.

Family Factors

To achieve relatively low mortality with substantial numbers of home births attended by TBAs or relatives, families need to be able to access emergency care when complications arise. Both the 1992 and 2000 studies show maternal deaths continue to occur because the woman and her family delay in seeking care. Delays complicate the management of the obstetrical emergencies at health facilities. As reported above, distance and lack of transport were rarely unavoidable factors. Therefore the reasons for referral delay or nonadherence with referral are more likely to be a lack of recognition of pregnancy danger signs and complications by women and their families, the attendants' lack of decisionmaking capacities regarding transfer, the judgment that health facilities are not of good quality, or the high cost (financially or socially) of complying with recommendations.

Studies in Egypt have highlighted the fact that many women cannot make autonomous decisions concerning their own health and must persuade other decisionmakers (the husband or mother-in-law) of the importance of their illnesses (Khattab 1992; Lane and Meleis 1991). The Egyptian demographic and health survey (EDHS) of 2000 indicates that 36 percent of women make decisions regarding their own health care by themselves and 24 percent make it jointly with their husbands or others. For 38 percent of women it is the husband alone who makes the decision and for 2 percent it is someone else (El Zanaty and Way 2001). Other studies have suggested that women's perceptions of poor quality services and financial costs are barriers to use of antenatal and delivery services, respectively (Loza 1994; SPAAC 1998).

Khattab (1992) identifies health professionals' lack of knowledge of the social conditions of women's lives as another reason for nonadherence. For example, a provider may tell a woman to get complete bed rest without checking whether this can be realistically managed. Women may also be told to take treatments they cannot afford. In addition, there is evidence that delay is still caused by the intermediate steps of women seeking care from private practitioners who were incapable of dealing with the medical emergency involved or who delayed transferring the women to higher-level facilities. As noted above, failure of the first medical provider to refer the woman was judged to have contributed to 13 percent of maternal deaths.

Mass-media health education campaigns have emphasized the need to seek medical care for life-threatening obstetric complications (MOH 1994; MotherCare Egypt Project 1998). More recently, in Upper Egypt, community efforts at outreach and cooperation with local providers have also tried to mobilize "birth preparedness" and community resources for such care (HM/HC RP

2000). Yet the EDHS 2000 shows that only 18 percent of women attending antenatal care were told about pregnancy danger signs and only 14 percent were told where to go if they had a complication. As there is no baseline information from earlier periods, however, it cannot be said that there has been a change in these family factors.

Other Policies Linked to Delivery Care

Conducting national confidential inquiries into maternal mortality in Egypt is a notable feat, and it appears that the 1992–93 NMMS, coupled with the international Safe Motherhood Initiative (Mahler 1987; Sai and Measham 1992; Starrs and the Inter-Agency Group for Safe Motherhood 1998), may have drawn attention to the magnitude of maternal deaths in Egypt and stimulated improvements. Many of the recommendations made in the 1992–93 report were adopted.

Antenatal Care

The effectiveness of antenatal care in preventing maternal death has been called into question (Maine 1991; Rooney 1992; Carroli, Rooney, and Villar 2001), especially the use of high-risk scoring systems with low predictive value. It is interesting to note that within the context of Egypt, maternal mortality had been nearly halved without a substantial increase in the percentage of women having antenatal care (see figure 6.3), although the percentage having more than four visits has increased. In nearly a fifth of maternal death cases, women attended antenatal care but had poor quality care. The percent of deceased women with no antenatal care slightly decreased from 35 percent in 1992–93 to 32 percent in 2000, whereas the percent with more than 10 visits increased from 13 percent in 1992–93 to 24 percent in 2000, possibly suggesting greater care seeking among women with complications. There has also been a tremendous increase in tetanus toxoid (TT) coverage, but this is unlikely to make a major contribution to maternal mortality (figure 6.4).

Figure 6.3 Egypt: Percentage of Pregnant Women with Antenatal Care; Percentage with 4+ Visits, 1976–2000

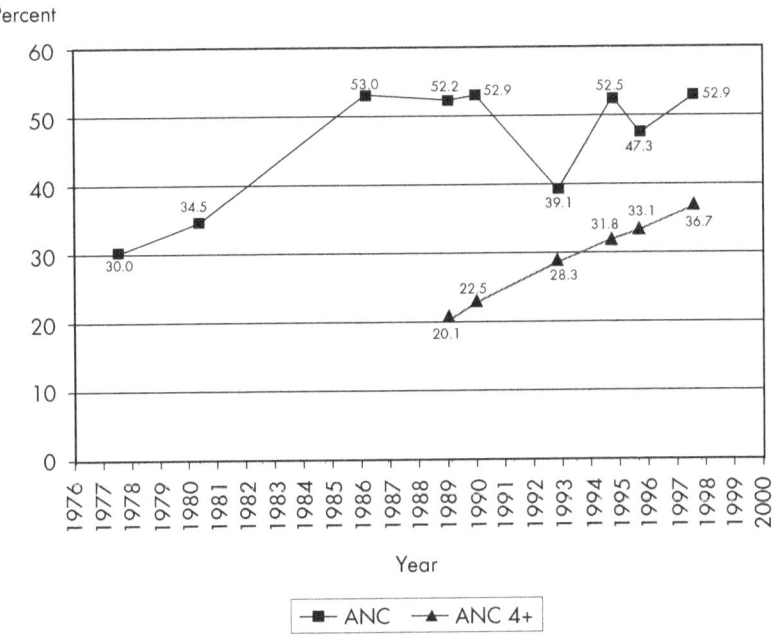

Note: ANC = antenatal care.
Source: El Zanaty and Way 2001; WHO 1988.

Fertility and Abortion

Egypt has made sustained efforts to reduce the fertility rate and unwanted births. Figure 6.5 shows national estimates of the contraceptive prevalence rate. The increased use of modern contraception from 23 percent in 1980 to 54 percent in 2000 and the decreasing total fertility rate from 5.3 in 1980 to 3.5 in 2000 (El-Zanaty and Way 2001) can affect maternal mortality in three ways. First, the number of pregnancies is reduced, thereby decreasing the number of times women face the risk of maternal death; second, high-risk pregnancies at higher parities can be avoided; and third, women can

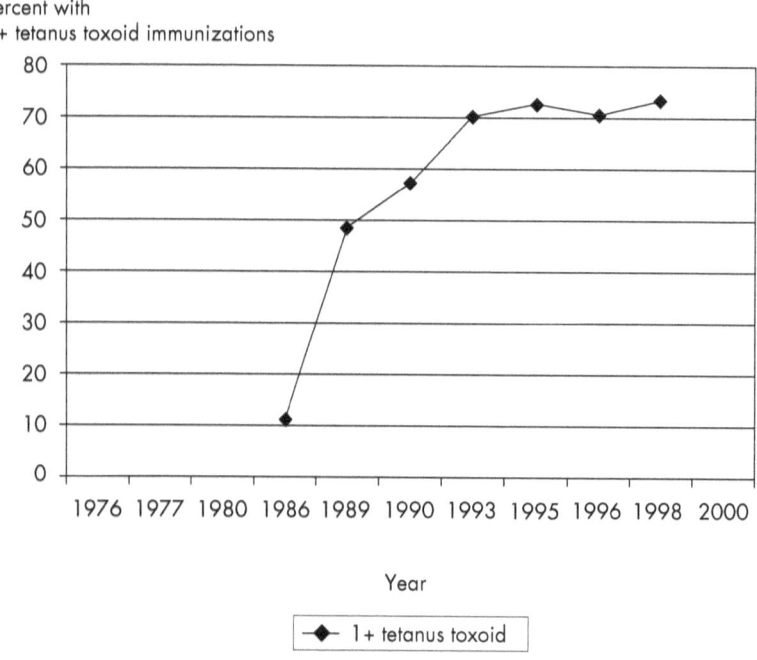

Figure 6.4 Egypt: Tetanus Toxoid Immunizations during Pregnancy, 1976–2000

Source: CAPMAS 1987; El-Zanaty and others 1995.

avoid unwanted pregnancy, which may end in illegally induced abortion or in poorer care-seeking behavior (Campbell and Graham 1990; Fortney 1987; Winikoff and Sullivan 1987). The biggest impact is likely to be through the first mechanism, though only the latter two are likely to affect the MMR.

In 1988, 24 percent of births were not wanted at all and 16 percent were wanted later (Sayed and others 1989), but by 2000, 13 percent of pregnancies were not wanted at all and 5 percent were wanted later. This suggests a big improvement in contraceptive access. In 85 percent of couples, both men and women approve of contraception (El-Zanaty and Way 2001). Among the maternal deaths in 2000, however, 6 percent had contraceptive failures and pregnancy was a serious problem in 10 percent of cases and a lesser problem in 7 percent of cases. According to the families, 22 percent of pregnancies were not wanted at all when they occurred and 5 percent were wanted later, indicating a missed opportunity for contraception.

Induced abortion is restricted to cases of life-threatening maternal health considerations and is surrounded by many social and religious sanctions. In the 2000 NMMS, induced abortions contributed to 2 percent of all maternal deaths, suggesting that induced abortion is not as large a problem in Egypt as in some other countries where

Figure 6.5 Egypt: Percentage of Women Using Modern Contraception, 1979–2001

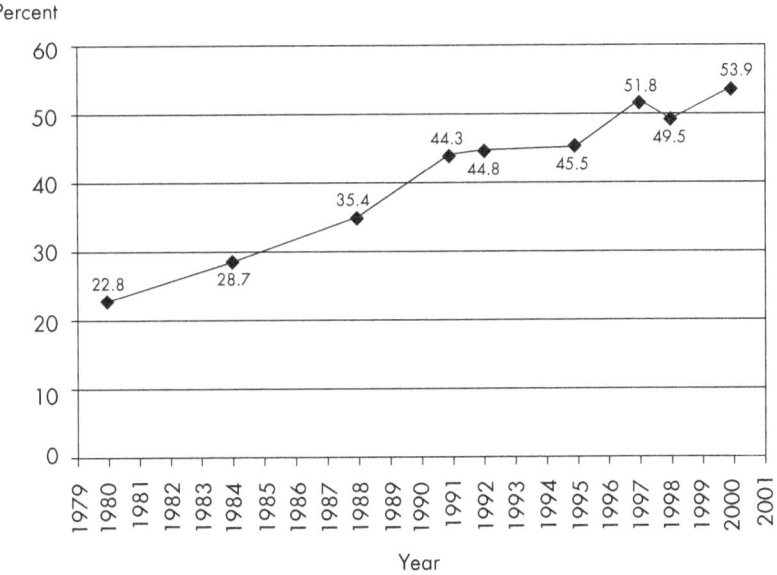

Sources: CAPMAS 1987; El-Zanaty and others 1993; El-Zanaty and others 1996; El-Zanaty and Way 2001.

it can contribute to over 50 percent of all maternal deaths (Royston and Armstrong 1989). El Mouelhy's (1987, 1992) data (including hospital admission case series) reported the proportion of all abortions that are induced or septic ranges from 2 to 60 percent, with a median of around 18 percent. Huntington and colleagues (1995) showed that standards in postabortion care in one large teaching facility in Cairo were poor but amenable to improvements.

Conclusion

Egypt has made good progress in reducing fertility and increasing access and use of skilled attendants and facility births. Some of the policies resulting in these changes did not appear to be specially developed for maternity care. However, further declines in maternal mortality ratios are likely to be contingent on taking a health systems approach and tackling health-system-wide problems (Goodburn and Campbell 2001). These include addressing linkages and continuity between antenatal, delivery, and postpartum care; strengthening referral systems; ensuring better oversight and regulation of the private sector; tackling deficiencies in hospital management and hospital systems; developing improved preservice training; elaborating mechanisms for updating inservice provider skills and knowledge; and strengthening accountability. In addition, because obstetricians are the predominant skilled attendants, careful attention needs to be given to avoiding overmedicalization and iatrogenic practice.

The Ministry of Health and Population also needs to conduct policy analyses for planning the future of delivery care. Important features are who should be delivering normal births and where should such births take place. In other words, Is the MOHP happy to encourage the trend of increased obstetrician deliveries, even if these were to reach 100 percent? What is the role of midwifery in Egypt, and should it be strengthened? Should births by skilled attendants take place in private clinics or in the public sector facilities? If in the public sector, should they be in hospitals, MCH units, other health centers with beds, or women's homes? What costs are associated with these options? To what extent should district hospitals be capable of EOC? Given the low volume in some of these hospitals, should resources be put into governorate hospitals instead? How can Egypt promote good evidence-based care among health facility births and avoid the overuse of practices such as augmentation, supine position, and lack of companionship (Chalmers, Enkin, and Keirse 1991; Enkin and others 1996)? Where would women like to deliver if resources were not a constraint?

References

Abdel-Azeem, F., S. M. Farid, and A. M. Khalifa. 1993. *Egypt Maternal and Child Health Survey 1991*. Pan Arab Project for Child Development. League of Arab States. Arab Republic of Egypt. CAPMAS.

Abdullah, S. A., E. M. Aboloyoun, H. Abdel-Aleem, F. M. Moftah, and S. Ismail. 1992. "Maternal Mortality in Assiut." *International Journal of Gynecology and Obstetrics* 39:197–204.

Abdullah, S. A., M. F. Fathalla, A. M. Abdel-Aleem, H. T. Salem, and M. Y. Aly. 1985. "Maternal Mortality in Upper Egypt." WHO Inter-Regional Meeting on Prevention of Maternal Mortality, November 11–15, Geneva.

Campbell, O. M. R., and W. J. Graham. 1990. "Measuring Maternal Mortality and Morbidity: Levels and Trends." Maternal and Child Epidemiology Unit Research Paper. London School of Hygiene and Tropical Medicine, London.

CAPMAS (Central Agency for Public Mobilization and Statistics). 1987. *Maternal Health and Infant Mortality in Egypt*. Cairo, Egypt.

Carroli, G., C. Rooney, and J. Villar. 2001. "How Effective Is Antenatal Care in Preventing Maternal Mortality and Serious Morbidity? An Overview of the Evidence." *Paediatric Perinatal Epidemiology* 15 (Suppl. 1):1–42.

Chalmers, Ian, M. Enkin, and M. J. N. C. Keirse. 1991. *Effective Care in Pregnancy and Childbirth*. Vols. 1 and 2. Oxford: Oxford University Press.

El Ghamry, A., et al. 1984. "The Feasibility of Getting Information about Maternal Mortality from the Husband." *Bulletin of the High Institute of Public Health* 14(2).

El Kady, A. A., S. Saleh, S. Gadalla, J. Fortney, and H. Bayoumi. 1989. "Obstetric Deaths in Menoufia Governorate, Egypt." *British Journal of Obstetrics and Gynaecology* 96:9–14.

El Mouelhy, M. T. 1987. *Maternal Mortality in Egypt*. Cairo Family Planning Association. Unpublished Report. Cairo, Egypt.

———. 1992. "Maternal Mortality in the Last Two Decades in Egypt." *Saudi Medical Journal* 13(2):132–36.

El-Zanaty, F. H., and A. A. Way. 2001. *Egypt Demographic Health Survey 2000*. Ministry of Health and Population, National Population Council, and ORC Macro.

El-Zanaty, F. H., N. Kumar, P. Berman, and W. Yip. 1995. "The Egyptian Household Health Care Utilization and Expenditure Survey, 1995." Annual Seminar on Population Issues in the Middle East, Africa and Asia, Cairo Demographic Centre. December 12–14. Cairo.

El-Zanaty, F. H., E. M. Hussein, G. A. Shawky, A. A. Way, and S. Kishor. 1996. "Final Report: Egypt (English) Survey Year: 1995." National Population Council and Macro International Inc.

El-Zanaty, F. H., H. A. A. Sayed, H. M. Zaky, and A. A. Way. 1993. "Final Report: Egypt (English) Survey Year: 1992." Egypt DHS 1992—Preliminary report. KZFR48. Cairo: Egypt National Population Council and Macro International Inc.

Enkin, M.W., M. J. N. C. Keirse, M. J. Renfrew, and J. P. Neilson, eds. 1996. "Pregnancy and Childbirth Module of The Cochrane Database of Systematic Reviews." The Cochrane Library, The Cochrane Collaboration, Issue 3. Oxford: Update Software.

Etman, Sayed, K. Omran, and J. Lewis. 1984. "Evaluation of TBA Program." In M. M. Fayed, I. I. Ibrahim, and M. A. Bayad, eds., *Medical Education in the Field of Primary Maternal Child Health Care*. Cairo: Cairo University Faculty of Medicine.

Fahmy, K. 1988. "Role of Training of Physicians in Improving Maternal Health from the University Point of View." In *Egyptian Society of Gynaecology and Obstetrics, and Egyptian Fertility Care Society Proceedings of the Safe Motherhood Conference, February 24–25*. Ismailia, Egypt: ESGO and EFCS.

Fortney, J. A. 1987. "The Importance of Family Planning in Reducing Maternal Mortality." *Studies in Family Planning* 18(2):109–14.

Fortney, J. A., S. Saleh, S. Gadalla, and S. M. Rogers. 1984. "Causes of Death to Women of Reproductive Age in Egypt." Working Papers in Development No. 49. Office of Women in International Development, Michigan State University, East Lansing.

Fortney, J. A., I. Susanti, S. Gadalla, S. Saleh, S. M. Rogers, and M. Potts. 1986. "Reproductive Mortality in Two Developing Countries." *American Journal of Public Health* 76:134–38.

Goodburn, Elizabeth, and O. Campbell. 2001. "Reducing Maternal Mortality in the Developing World: Sector-Wide Approaches May Be the Key." *British Medical Journal* 322(7291):917–20.

Hefni, M. M., and F. Kassas. 1991. "Daya Training Program, Part I." UNICEF Egypt Working Paper, August 1985. Cairo, Egypt.

HM/HC RP (Healthy Mother/Healthy Child Results Package). 2000. *HEALTHY MOTHER/HEALTHY CHILD 2000.* Briefing book. Cairo: John Snow, Inc.

Huntington, Dale, E. O. Hassan, N. Attallah, N. Toubia, M. Naguib, and L. Nawar. 1995. "Improving the Medical Care and Counseling of Post Abortion Patients in Egypt. *Studies in Family Planning* 26(6):350–62.

Khattab, H. A. S. 1992. *The Silent Endurance: Social Conditions of Women's Reproductive Health in Rural Egypt.* Cairo: UNICEF.

Lane, S. D., and A. I. Meleis. 1991. "Roles, Work, Health Perceptions and Health Resources of Women: A Study in an Egyptian Delta Hamlet." *Social Science and Medicine* 33(10):1197–208.

Loza, S. 1994. "Child Survival: Further Analysis of Baseline KAP Findings." Draft Report. Egypt: Social Planning Analysis and Administration Consultants.

Mahler, Halfden. 1987. "The Safe Motherhood Initiative: A Call to Action." *Lancet* 668–70.

Maine, Deborah. 1991. *Safe Motherhood Programs: Options and Issues.* Center for Population and Family Health, School of Public Health, Faculty of Medicine. New York: Columbia University.

MOH (Ministry of Health). 1994. *National Maternal Mortality Study: Egypt 1992–1993.* Preliminary report of findings and conclusions. Cairo: Child Survival Project.

MOHP (Ministry of Health and Population). 1997. "Rapid Assessment for the Maternal Mortality in Egypt." Esmat Mansour (General Director for Maternal and Child Health Care and Executive Director for Healthy Mother/Health Child Project); Said El Sharkawy (Consultant for HM/HC project).

———. 2000. *Basic Essential Obstetric Care Service Standards: Protocols for Physicians.* Cairo, Egypt.

———. 2001. *National Maternal Mortality Study: Egypt 2000.* Preliminary report of findings and conclusions. Cairo: Child Survival Project.

———. no date. *Essential Obstetric Care and Neonatal Care. Community Development, Planning and Management.* The Maternal and Child Health series. Cairo, Egypt.

MotherCare Egypt Project. 1998. *The Final Report, September 1996–1998.* Ministry of Health and Population. Healthy Mother Healthy Child Project. Cairo. Contract No. HRN-5966-Q-00-3039-0.

Ricter, Anne. 1992. *Daya Training Programme Evaluation: May 1992.* Cairo: Ministry of Health Child Survival Project, Child Spacing Component.

Rooney, C. I. F. 1992. "Antenatal Care and Maternal Health: How Effective Is It?" Document WHO/MSM/92.4. Geneva: World Health Organization.

Royston, Erica, and S. Armstrong. 1989. *Preventing Maternal Deaths.* Geneva: World Health Organization.

Sai, F. T., and D. M. Measham. 1992. "Safe Motherhood Initiative: Getting Our Priorities Straight." *Lancet* 339:478–80.

Saleh, S., S. Gadalla, J. A. Fortney, and S. Morsy, eds. 1987. "Maternal Mortality in Menoufia: A Study of Reproductive Age Mortality." Cairo: Social Research Center, American University.

Sallam, I. 1998. "Health Care in Egypt" (letter). *Lancet* 352(9140):1632.

Sayed, H. A. A. 1991. *Egypt Service Availability Survey 1989: Availability and Accessibility of Family Planning and Health Services in Rural Egypt.* Columbia, Md.: Cairo Demographic Centre and Demographic and Health Surveys and IRD Macro International Inc.

Sayed, H. A. A., M. I. Osman, F. El-Zanaty, and A. A. Way. 1989. *Egypt Demographic and Health Survey 1988.* Final Report: Egypt (English). Columbia, Md.: Institute for Resource Development/Macro Systems, Inc.

SPAAC (Social Planning Analysis and Administration Consultants). 1998. *MotherCare Egypt Diagnostic Research in the Governorate of Aswan and Luxor: Final Report.* Cairo, Egypt.

Stanton, Cynthia, N. Abderrahim, and K. Hill. 1997. *DHS Maternal Mortality Indicators: An Assessment of Data Quality and Implications for Data Use.* DHS Analytical Reports No. 4 Calverton, Md.: Macro International Inc.

Starrs, Anne, and the Inter-Agency Group for Safe Motherhood. 1998. *The Safe Motherhood Action Agenda: Priorities for the Next Decade.* New York: Family Care International.

UNICEF (United Nations Children's Fund). 1985. *Daya Training Programme in Egypt.* Cairo: UNICEF.

Winikoff, Beverly, and M. Sullivan. 1987. "Assessing the Role of Family Planning in Reducing Maternal Mortality." *Studies in Family Planning* 18:128–42.

WHO (World Health Organization, Division of Family Health). 1988. *Coverage of Maternity Care: A Tabulation of Available Information,* 1st ed. Geneva: WHO.

———. 1993. *Coverage of Maternity Care: A Tabulation of Available Information,* 3rd ed. Geneva: WHO.

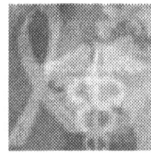

CHAPTER 7

Indonesia, 1990–1999
Marjorie A. Koblinsky

The fourth most populous country in the world, with a high MMR of 334 per 100,000 live births (second only to Cambodia within the Association of Southeast Asian Nations region), Indonesia suffers death from childbirth of approximately 22,000 women each year (CBS and others 1998). To address this problem, the country embraced a recommendation of the Safe Motherhood Initiative—a skilled attendant at each birth—as the likeliest way to reduce pregnancy-related mortality and morbidity. The government decided that the skilled attendant should be a certified midwife placed in each village. Although Indonesia had phased out its midwifery schools in 1975, neighboring Malaysia had met with success in reducing its MMR after initiating a strategy with village-based midwives in the 1950s. So in 1989, the Indonesian Safe Motherhood Initiative was launched by the president, who stated at the time that there should be one midwife per village to reduce the MMR (or one midwife per 1,000 population, with approximately 23 births a year).

Prior to this new policy, much of the government's focus had been on training TBAs and on the provision of preventive activities for mothers and children at the monthly village sessions staffed by the local health center, the *posyandu*. Here antenatal care and family planning for women were joined with preventive services for children—immunizations, nutrition, and diarrhea control. Programmatic thinking of 1989–90 focused on partnering the TBA with the health center staff at a *polindes*, a community-constructed hut where births could take place with both TBAs and health center midwives (*bidans*) present. However, less than 1 percent of births took place in the polindes, even five years later (CBS and others 1998), primarily because they were little more than a TBA-assisted birth at greater cost and with far less support than offered in the home.

Increased Availability

To fulfill the presidential decree, officials determined that 54,000 midwives needed to be trained, with the first batch available for village-level service by 1993. To prepare the village midwives (*bidan di desa*, or BDD), training consisted of three years of nursing, followed by one year of midwifery. Cost of this training was approximately US$1,800 per village midwife (Hull, Rusman, and Hayes 1999). Following training, they were posted to the village—with little preparation for community work yet with the understanding that they were to develop their own support within three years. (The government initially provided them with a three-year contract for service; it later gave them a second three-year contract.)

With the BDD program ongoing, the government phased out any TBA training where BDDs were posted. Even so the 1998 DHS showed that 68 percent of births still took place in women's homes; 11 percent occurred at bidans' homes or someone else's, 12 percent in private facilities, and only 9 percent in government facilities. Hospital use has not increased significantly since the BDD program began, moving from 5.7 to 6.2 percent (public hospitals) and from 4.9 to 4.7 percent for private hospitals between 1994 and 1997 (CBS and others 1995; CBS and others 1998). The birth attendant has slightly shifted over this same time frame, with the bidan (including BDD) assistance for birthing increasing from 35 percent in 1994 to 44 percent in 1997, displacing the TBA, who, however, still provided birth attendance for over 45 percent of deliveries in 1997 (table 7.1). Hence Indonesia is in the process of shifting from a Model 1 setting to Model 2, but the placement of village midwives close to women did not automatically result in Model 2.

Table 7.1 Indonesia: Assistance during Delivery, 1990, 1994, and 1997 (percent)

YEAR	DOCTOR	TRAINED NURSE MIDWIFE OR OTHER HEALTH PROFESSIONAL	TRADITIONAL BIRTH ATTENDANT	RELATIVE OR OTHER	NO ONE	DATA MISSING	TOTAL
1990	4.9	30.9	59.6	4.4	0.3	0	100.0
1994	6.7	34.8	54.4	3.7	0.4	0	100.0
1997	7.4	43.6	46.1	2.7	0.2	0	100.0

Sources: CBS and others 1991, 1995, 1998.

Competence of Provider

Communities were prepared for neither the services of the village midwives nor the need to pay for those services. Problems ensued, ranging from poor quality of services and low retention rates, especially in the remoter areas, to low demand rates for the midwives' maternity services. Looking specifically at elements that contribute to quality of care, village midwives less than three years from training could correctly address less than 60 percent of questions on a knowledge test in a MotherCare project in South Kalimantan. Their confidence in performing their midwifery skills was also low—less than 60 percent. Performance of specific skills (such as infection prevention, use of the partograph, bimanual compression, manual removal of the placenta, and neonatal resuscitation) was on average 51 percent (percent mean score), with neonatal resuscitation and bimanual compression both less than 40 percent (figure 7.1). Only 6 percent of the village midwives tested scored 70 percent or higher in these skills, a level considered to be needed for competence (McDermott and others 2001). Facility-based midwives who had been practicing for many years more than the village midwives also scored poorly. Their scores in both knowledge of what to do and confidence in performing specific tasks (in infection prevention and antenatal, delivery, and postpartum care) were less than 50 percent and a skills assessment gave a mean score of 40 percent for these experienced bidans.

Figure 7.1 South Kalimantan, Indonesia: Skill Scores for Midwives by Procedures, 1999

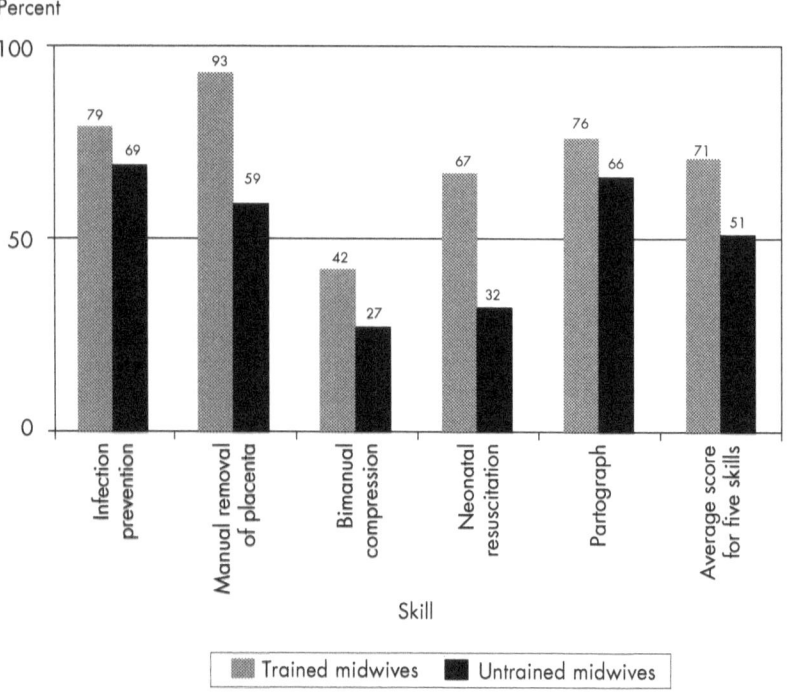

Source: McDermott and others 2001.

When both village and facility-based midwives were provided with a two-week competency-based training course in some lifesaving skills, their skills increased significantly: 67 percent and 46 percent, respectively, achieved competency compared with 6 percent and 0 percent for unretrained midwives, as figure 7.2 shows (McDermott and others 2001). To raise the midwife's skills to competency level costs approximately US$253 per village midwife and US$320 per facility-based midwife (table 7.2); these are costs of expansion, minus start-up, technical assistance, and central administrative costs (Walker and others 2002).

Figure 7.2 South Kalimantan, Indonesia: Skill Scores and Competency for Midwives by Groups, 1999

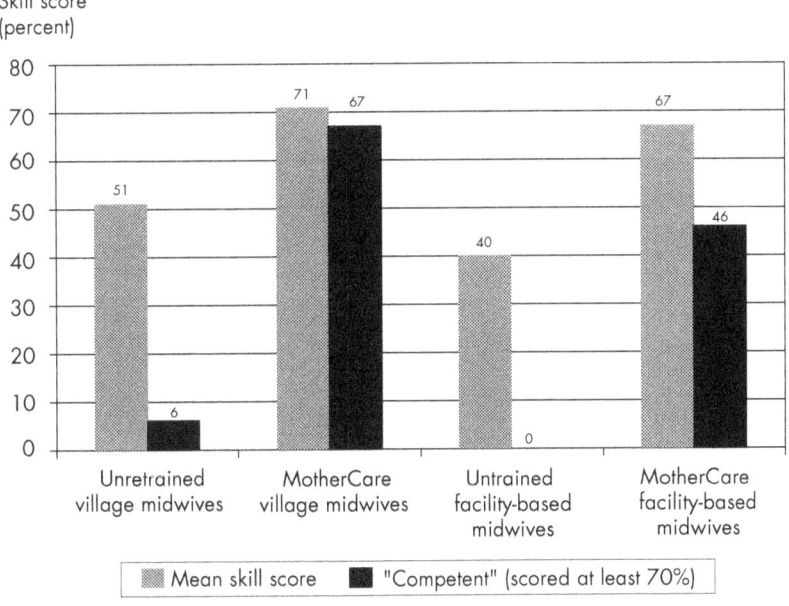

Source: McDermott and others 2001.

Table 7.2 South Kalimantan, Indonesia: Costs of Training Programs, 1999

INDICATOR	MOTHERCARE TRAINING PROGRAMS	
	FACILITY MIDWIFE	VILLAGE MIDWIFE
Total cost (US$)	$147,704	$344,774
Number of trainees	110	284
Cost per trainee (US$)	$1,343	$1,214
Cost per trainee—replication (US$)	$512	$384
Cost per trainee—expansion (US$)	$320	$253

Source: Walker and others 2002.

Improving Safe Motherhood in South Kalimantan

Given a package of interventions in South Kalimantan that included not only the training of midwives, but also a communications strategy to alert women and families of the need to use midwives' services, especially for delivery, and a districtwide maternal-perinatal audit, the use of midwives for birth did increase. Between 1993 and 1996, the majority (90 percent) of births took place at home in South Kalimantan, and skilled attendants (doctors or midwives) attended only 37 percent of all births (home and facility). By 1998–99, 510 midwives were posted in the three project districts, and skilled attendance at delivery had increased to 59 percent ($p = 0.0003$). However, the proportion delivering at home remained stable at 88 percent of births ($p = 0.3$). There was no increase in the use of hospitals for delivery. Ronsmans and her coauthors (2001) conclude that costs of care may be a major constraining factor on use of hospital care, along with lack of transport and lack of cultural acceptability.

Costs as a Barrier

In 1996 women in South Kalimantan reported a median expenditure of Rp 600,000 (US$240) for a cesarean section. This is approximately one-fifth of the average GDP per capita for Indonesia for that year (GDP 1996 = $1,136). Minimum fees for a cesarean section remained stable over the study period, although the economic crises beginning in 1997 stretched household funds. Between 1997 and 1999, the proportion of hospitalized women relying on a certificate giving free access to care increased from 1.5 to 11.4 percent. Despite this, the proportion admitted to hospital for cesarean section (from admissions records and population birthrates) declined from 1.7 to 1.4 percent ($p = 0.005$). Similarly the proportion admitted to hospital with a complication requiring a lifesaving intervention declined from 1.1 to 0.7 percent ($p = 0.001$) (Ronsmans and others 2001). Trends were consistent across districts (see figures 7.3 and 7.4).

Figure 7.3 South Kalimantan, Indonesia: Proportion of Cesarean Sections among Births, 1997–99

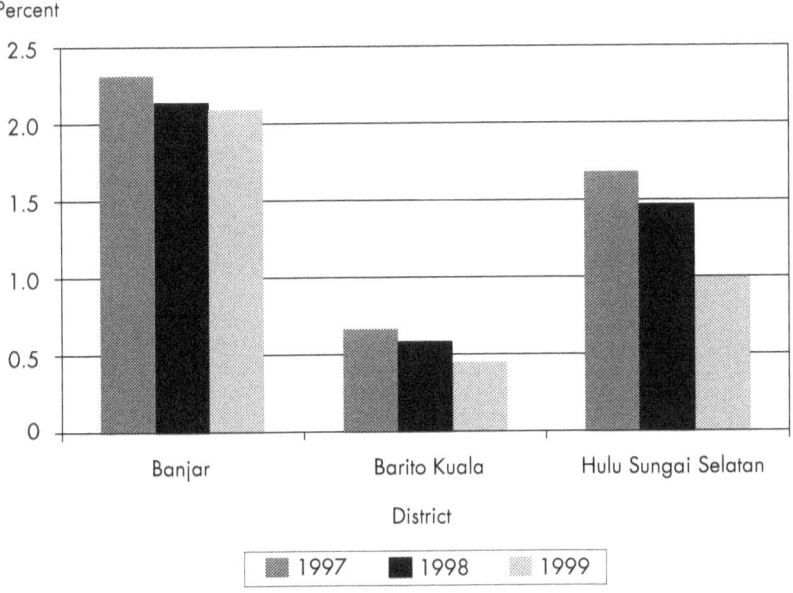

Source: Ronsmans and others 2001.

Conclusion

The strategy of a midwife in every village has clearly resulted in a dramatic increase in skilled birth attendance, but not as yet in any increase in specialized obstetric care for the women needing it. Although the midwives may have treated more complications at home, it is unlikely that they could have prevented or treated most of the severe complications that require a major hospital intervention to save the woman's life. Despite the government's efforts to overcome financial constraints for the poor during the economic crisis, the high costs of emergency obstetric interventions may well have remained the most important obstacle to use of hospital care.

The last BDD cohort that will enjoy the maximum of two three-year contracts after graduating is the one trained in 1999, meaning

Figure 7.4 South Kalimantan, Indonesia: Proportion of Births with Life-Threatening Complications in the Hospital, 1997–99

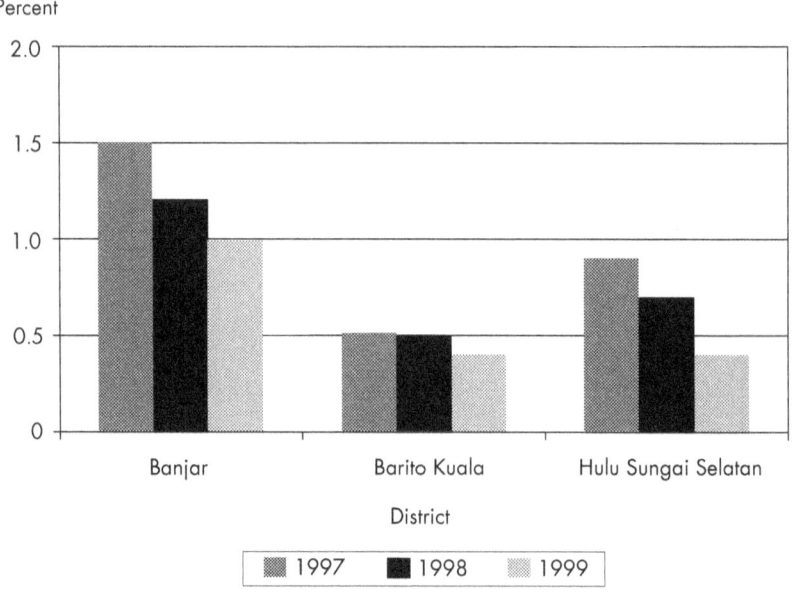

Source: Ronsmans and others 2001.

government support for the BDD program will end in 2005. Beyond the costs of hospital care, another major challenge is the sustainability of the village midwife program as the country begins the transition to decentralized governance initiated in mid-2001. Whether the seat of authority for health will be at the district level or shared between the district, province, and central levels, the priority, and hence survival, of the BDD program is likely to be determined at a more local level. Issues of quality of care, supervision, immediate authority, continued bifurcation of family planning and maternity care, and integration of the services at the three levels of care (hospitals, health centers, and community) remain and will have to be addressed by whomever is in charge. Yet resources throughout the country have become strained since the economic crisis began in 1997, meaning private sources of funding will become more important—and perhaps scarcer—for many programs, including the BDD program.

References

CBS (Central Bureau of Statistics) (Indonesia), NFPCB (State Ministry of Population/National Family Planning Coordinating Board), MOH (Ministry of Health), and MI (Macro International Inc.). 1991. *Indonesia Demographic and Health Survey, 1990.* Calverton, Md.: CBS and MI.

———. 1995. *Indonesia Demographic and Health Survey, 1994.* Calverton, Md.: CBS and MI.

———. 1998. *Indonesia Demographic and Health Survey, 1997.* Calverton, Md.: CBS and MI.

Hull, T. H., R. Rusman, and A. C. Hayes. 1999. *Village Midwives and the Improvement of Maternal and Infant Health in Nusa Tenggara Timur and Nusa Tenggara Barat.* Report. Australian Agency for International Development, Sidney, Australia.

McDermott, Jeanne, D. Beck, S. T. Buffington, J. Anna, and G. Supratikto. 2001. "Two Models of In-Service Training to Improve Midwifery Skills: How Well Do They Work?" *Journal of Midwifery & Women's Health* 46(4):217–25.

Ronsmans, Carine, E. Achadi, S. Gunawan, A. Zazri, J. McDermott, M. Koblinsky, and T. Marshall. 2001. "Evaluation of a Comprehensive Home-Based Midwifery Programme in South Kalimantan, Indonesia." *Tropical Medicine and International Health* 6(10):799–810.

Walker, Damien, J. M. McDermott, J. Fox-Rushby, M. Tanjung, M. Nadjib, D. Widiatmoko, and E. Achadi. 2002. "An Economic Analysis of a Midwifery Training Programme in South Kalimantan, Indonesia." *WHO Bulletin* 80(1):47–55.

CHAPTER 8

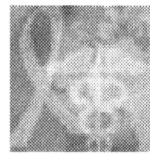

Jamaica, 1991–1995
Affete McCaw-Binns

From 1938 to 1960 the MMR in Jamaica decreased from 600 to 210 per 100,000 live births (Williams 1973). By 1981–83 it had decreased further to 108 (Walker and others 1986), where it essentially remained for the next few years, being reported as 115 in a 1986–87 study (Keeling and others 1991).

Between 1981 and 1983, approximately 72 percent of all births occurred in health institutions (Walker and others 1990). In 1986–87, midwives attended 75 percent of deliveries; doctors and medical students attended only 9 percent (Figueroa, Ashley, and McCaw-Binns 1990). The same survey found that untrained midwives attended 5 percent of deliveries, while no one attended 8 percent. Hence, by the 1980s most Jamaican women were in a Model 3 or 4 setting.

The 1986–87 nationwide study reported 62 maternal deaths: 19 (31 percent) died from hypertension, 15 (24 percent) from hemorrhage, 11 (18 percent) from infection, and 17 (27 percent) from other causes. The major cause of death, hypertension, had also been the primary cause of maternal death in the 1981–83 study. Almost all women in this category in the 1986–87 study died as a result of eclamptic fits.

Geographic access to care had been a major barrier for the women who died. Jamaica is divided into 14 administrative sectors (parishes). Three contain type A hospitals (tertiary obstetrical care) and four have type B (specialist obstetric and pediatric services), but half have only type C facilities (basic maternal, general medical, and surgical services) (Golding and others 1989). There is a network of

364 primary health care centers that provide only basic antenatal, postnatal, child health care, curative, and domiciliary midwifery services. Of the 19 hypertensive deaths in 1986–87, 12 (63 percent) were delivered at a type C hospital or at home. Similarly, 10 of the 11 hemorrhage deaths, and 6 of the 8 infection deaths, also occurred among women who delivered in a type C facility or at home (Keeling and others 1991).

Addressing the Major Killer

To address the high rate of eclampsia deaths, health officials developed a pilot project in one parish to ensure that primary care antenatal clinics had clear instructions for referring patients to a high-risk clinic or straight to a hospital. Clear guidelines were also provided for action at the high-risk clinics and referral hospital, detailing when induction of labor should occur and the appropriate treatment for hypertension and preeclampsia.

The parish of St. Catherine, with its 7,000 deliveries per year, was chosen for the study, which took place between 1992 and 1995. This parish has one type C and one type B hospital. St. Ann and Manchester were chosen as control parishes, each with one type B hospital and an urban-rural mix similar to that of the intervention area. In the intervention parish, clear guidelines for identification of high-risk women were prepared for the midwives who carried out antenatal care. The only equipment provided was variable-width cuffs and Uristix for testing urine for protein. Public health nurses, community midwives, and community health aides were trained to identify and follow up women at risk of developing hypertension. An "intervention" nurse visited all health centers to help the frontline midwives use the monitoring tools and distribute supplies. Frequent meetings were held with midwives to feed back information to staff and facilitate the exchange of information between primary- and secondary-care levels to solve problems. Private practitioners were also given information to ensure early referral of women with signs of hypertension or preeclampsia. At the type B hospital, all members

Table 8.1 Jamaica: Odds Ratio of Antenatal Eclampsia Cases—Intervention Parish Compared with Control Parishes, 1986–95

YEAR	INTERVENTION	CONTROL	ODDS RATIO
1986–91	84	50	1.00 reference
1992	13	9	0.86 (0.34, 2.15)
1993	11	10	0.66 (0.26, 1.66)
1994	8	13	0.37 (0.14, 0.95)
1995	4	13	0.18 (0.06, 0.58)

Note: $p < 0.001$ trend.
Source: McCaw-Binns and others 2000.

of the nursing staff received training as they rotated among the services. The consultant obstetricians were enthusiastic and often participated in discussions.

All referred patients had to be seen by an obstetrician at a high-risk clinic; three such clinics were set up in St. Catherine to ensure short waiting times and the presence of an obstetrician. All patients with diastolic blood pressure 100 mm Hg or more were given antihypertensive therapy. Magnesium sulphate or Diazepam was administered if eclampsia seemed imminent. Labor was induced with misoprostol. Women were given information directly by means of posters and booklets.

Results

Table 8.1 shows the numbers of cases of antenatal eclampsia in the 10 years from 1986 to 1995. It can be seen that in the control areas, there was an increasing trend for antepartum eclampsia to occur, whereas in the intervention area, starting in 1992, a decrease in eclampsia occurred ($p < 0.001$). There were no changes in the total number of births in each area that could explain this (McCaw-Binns and others 2000).

The total number of admissions per year for hypertensive disorders of pregnancy before the intervention was 252; this dropped to 150 after the intervention (table 8.2). Bed days for women with

Table 8.2 Jamaica: Number of Bed Days Used by Mothers Admitted for the Hypertensive Disorders of Pregnancy before and at the End of the Intervention Period, 1991–95

CONDITION	INDICATOR	BEFORE (1991)	AFTER (1995)
Mild/moderate	No. admitted per year	170	105
	No. bed days per year	1,498	755[a]
	Bed days/admission	8.81 (+/−7.35)	7.19 (+/−6.24)
Severe preeclampsia	No. admitted per year	36	30 n.s.
	No. bed days per year	398	206[a]
	Bed days/admission	11.06 (+/−6.27)	6.85 (+/−3.66)
Eclampsia	No. admitted per year	13	4[b]
	No. bed days per year	108	20[a]
	Bed days/admission	8.31 (+/−4.05)	5.00 (+/−3.16)
All hypertension-related admissions	No. admitted per year	252	150[a]
	No. bed days per year	2,255	1,038[a]
	Bed days/admission	8.95 (+/−7.10)	6.92 (+/−5.54)

n.s. Not statistically significant.
a. $p < 0.0001$.
b. $p < 0.05$.
Source: McCaw-Binns and others 2000.

hypertension were 2,255 in the year before the intervention began, and they declined to 1,038 in the last year of the intervention.

The number of admissions for eclampsia fell dramatically (from 13 to 4), with a consequent drop in the number of bed days used for eclampsia from 108 to 20. The admission numbers for women with severe preeclampsia did not change over time, but duration of stay declined to 6.85 days on average from 11 days. Comparison for mild preeclampsia showed 170 admissions per year preintervention to 105 postintervention. Although the stay per admission remained at 7 days compared with the earlier duration of 8.8 days, total bed days declined from 1,498 in 1990 to only 755 at the end of the study period.

Before intervention women with hypertensive disorders occupied about six beds per day; after the intervention fewer than three beds per day were so occupied. In the control areas no change occurred. Costs of the intervention (training, setting up the high-risk clinics, hiring an intervention nurse, and distributing cuffs and supplies) have been offset by the reduction in bed days for hypertensive disorders.

Improving Demand

Noting that problems still remained with referral after the first intervention study, MacGillivray went on to develop and test a mother-held card identifying six particular signs and symptoms of hypertension that should be acted upon by immediately going to the health center or local midwife. These were frontal headache, epigastric pain, dimness of vision or seeing spots or flashes, edema, vomiting during the last trimester of pregnancy, and antepartum hemorrhage (another problem for which women should seek care; not related to pregnancy-induced hypertension). The card was to be given to women during their first antenatal care visit. A poster with similar messages was hung in all primary- and secondary-care antenatal clinics. Selected for the trial was St. Ann's parish, which had 3,500 births annually and high eclampsia rates that seemed to be on the rise.

The cards and posters increased awareness among the mothers as well as the midwives in the antenatal clinics. Awareness among mothers who had not seen the card was 67 percent in response to the question of what they would do if "your feet were swollen and it was uncomfortable to walk." After the intervention, awareness of signs of hypertension was 92 percent among those who had seen the poster and been given a card. Of the women who had received a card and responded positively that they had suffered one of the signs or symptoms depicted on the card, only 7 of 134 mothers reported having taken no action. Eclampsia also decreased in the area—from 8.1 cases over a 10-month period to 3 cases in this time frame. Just how much the cards and posters decreased the eclampsia rate is unknown, but certainly they are associated with the increased awareness.

Conclusion

Using a very targeted approach to reduce one of the primary direct causes of maternal mortality required specific training with frontline providers. It also required training of those who support the midwife, linking the levels of care with a high-risk clinic to manage cases, and linking with the private physicians so that referrals from the private sector increased to 44 percent (the rest of the island is 20 percent). In order to ensure that women themselves knew the danger signs and where to seek care, health officials provided them with a card alerting them to the danger signs. This has been well used by them to initiate appropriate care.

Did this targeted intervention have an impact on maternal deaths? In St. Catherine there were 12 maternal deaths in 1986 (4 eclampsia or hypertension related); for 1993, 1994, and 1995, there were 8 (3 eclampsia), 9 (2 eclampsia), and 7 maternal deaths (4 eclampsia), respectively. Eclampsia deaths had declined during the intervention period, but obviously managing care and ensuring that women come for care early and go to the hospital or high-risk clinic when advised need constant reinforcement to continue to have an impact (McCaw-Binns, personal communication, 2002).

References

Figueroa, J. P., D. Ashley, and A. McCaw-Binns. 1990. "An Evaluation of the Domiciliary Midwifery Services in Jamaica." *West Indian Medical Journal* 39:91–98.

Golding, Jean, D. Ashley, A. McCaw-Binns, J. W. Keeling, and T. Shenton. 1989. "Maternal Mortality in Jamaica: Socioeconomic Factors." *Acta Obstetrica Gynaecologica Scandanavica* 687:581–87.

Keeling, J. W., A. McCaw-Binns, D. Ashley, and J. Golding. 1991. "Maternal Mortality in Jamaica: Health Care Provision and Causes of Death." *International Journal of Gynecology and Obstetrics* 35:19–27.

MacGillivray, Ian, A. McCaw-Binns, D. Ashley, A. Fedrick, and J. Golding. 2000. "Strategies to Prevent Eclampsia in a Developing Country II, Use of a Pictorial Card." Final Report. Department of Community Health and Psychiatry, University of the West Indies, Mona, Jamaica.

McCaw-Binns, Affete, D. Ashley, L. Knight, I. MacGillivray, and J. Golding. 2000. "Strategies to Prevent Eclampsia in a Developing Country, Reorganization of Maternity Services." Final Report. Department of Community Health and Psychiatry, University of the West Indies, Mona, Jamaica.

Walker, G. J. A., A. McCaw-Binns, D. Ashley, and G. Bernard. 1986. "Maternal Mortality in Jamaica." *Lancet* 1(8479):486–88.

———. 1990. "Identifying Maternal Deaths in Developing Countries: Experience in Jamaica." *International Journal of Epidemiology* 19(3):599–605.

Williams, L. L. 1973. "Some Observations on Maternal Mortality in Jamaica." *West Indian Medical Journal* 22(1):1–18.

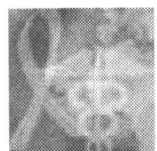

Contributors

Juan Carlos Arraya
MotherCare/John Snow, Inc. Research and Training Institute, Bolivia

Oona Campbell
London School of Hygiene and Tropical Medicine

Isabella Danel
The World Bank

Ramiro Equiluz
MotherCare/John Snow, Inc. Research and Training Institute, Bolivia

Shinga Feresu
University of Zimbabwe

Institute for Health Science
Kunming Medical College, Yunnan, China

Marjorie A. Koblinsky
John Snow, Inc. Research and Training Institute, Washington, D.C.
North American Consortium for IMMPACT,
Bloomberg School of Public Health, Johns Hopkins University

Leonard Mumbwanda
Ministry of Health, Zimbabwe

Margaret Nyandoro
Ministry of Health, Zimbabwe

Guillermo Seoane
MotherCare/John Snow, Inc. Research and Training Institute, Bolivia

Affete McCaw-Binns
University of the West Indies, Jamaica

Ada Rivera
Ministry of Health, Honduras

Miguel Ugalde
MotherCare/John Snow, Inc. Research and Training Institute, Bolivia

www.ingramcontent.com/pod-product-compliance
Lightning Source LLC
Chambersburg PA
CBHW022013160426
43197CB00007B/413